Multipl
Questio
Radiodi

CW0072527Ø

Ann Crozier MBChB DMRD FRCR
Consultant Radiologist, Glenfield Hospital, Leicester

David Finlay MBChB MRCP(UK) DMRD FRCR DCH
Consultant Radiologist, Leicester Royal Infirmary,
Leicester

Paula Paciorek MBChB DMRD FRCR
Consultant Radiologist, The William Harvey Hospital,
Willesborough, Kent

Churchill Livingstone
EDINBURGH LONDON MELBOURNE AND NEW YORK 1986

Preface

This book contains multiple choice questions in radiodiagnosis. It is intended for those preparing for the final examination in diagnostic radiology. The questions are chosen to cover the field of knowledge required, and are designed to provide teaching as well as practice in answering multiple choice questions.

The questions are divided into ten papers of thirty questions each.

Each question should be answered by deciding true or false for each item.

We gratefully acknowledge assistance from Dr P Ander, J Berry, J Davies and Christine Reek. Our thanks also to Miss R Sutton and Mrs L Sewart for their secretarial assistance.

Ann Crozier
David Finlay
Paula Paciorek

CHURCHILL LIVINGSTONE
Medical Division of Longman Group UK Limited

Distributed in the United States of America by Churchill
Livingstone Inc., 1560 Broadway, New York, N.Y. 10036,
and by associated companies, branches and representatives
throughout the world.

First published 1986

ISBN 0 443 03692 6

British Library Cataloguing in Publication Data
Crozier, Ann
    Multiple choice questions in radiodiagnosis.
    —(MCQs)
    1. Diagnosis, Radioscopic—Problems,
    exercises, etc.
    I. Title   II. Finlay, David   III. Paciorek,
    Paula
    616.07'57'076   RC78

Library of Congress Cataloging-in-Publication Data
Crozier, Ann.
    Multiple choice questions in radiodiagnosis.
    Bibliography: p.
    1. Diagnosis, Radioscopic — Examinations, questions,
etc. I. Finlay, D. B. L. (David B. L.) II. Paciorek,
Paula. III. Title. [DNLM: 1. Radiography — examination
questions. WN 18 C954m]
RC78.15.C76   1986   616.07'57'076   86-17162

Produced by Longman Singapore Publishers (Pte) Ltd.
Printed in Singapore

Contents

Contents

A

Questions

A1 Partial absence of a clavicle has been described in
(a) trisomy 17–18
(b) Wegener's granulomatosis
(c) cleidocranial dysostosis
(d) rheumatoid arthritis
(e) osteogenesis imperfecta

A2 Carcinoma of the oesophagus is associated with
(a) ectopic columnar cell mucosa
(b) previous ingestion of corrosives
(c) tylosis
(d) epidermiolysis bullosa
(e) dermatomyositis

A3 When there is an injury in the lower leg
(a) diastasis at the ankle joint is occasionally associated with a spiral fracture in the proximal quarter of the fibula
(b) stress fractures of the distal fibula occur characteristically in ballet dancers
(c) osteochondral fractures of the dome of the talus are associated with eversion injuries of the ankle joint
(d) oblique fractures of the medial malleolus are associated with impaction of the talus
(e) tear of the lateral ankle ligament can be demonstrated by peroneal tenography

A4 Haemochromatosis
(a) is inherited as autosomal dominant
(b) commonly involves the hip joint
(c) commonly caused calcification of the triangular cartilage of the wrist
(d) is associated with sodium pyrophosphate crystals in synovial fluid
(e) causes increased density of liver on computerised tomographic scan of the abdomen

A5 On a computerised tomographic examination of the adrenals
(a) lesions as small as 0.5 cm can be visualised

(b) phaeochromocytomas sometimes show areas of low density
(c) adenomas can be differentiated from neuroblastoma
(d) metastatic lesions commonly arise from the ovary
(e) the normal contour of the glands is lost in bilateral hyperplasia

A6 Renal calculi are associated with
(a) *Proteus* infections
(b) congenital cyanotic heart disease
(c) polycythaemia
(d) hereditary spherocytosis
(e) horseshoe kidney

A7 The following are features of spinal dysraphism:
(a) abnormally high termination of the spinal cord
(b) widening of the spinal canal
(c) lipoma within the spinal canal
(d) pilonidal sinus
(e) neuroenteric cyst

A8 The following are correct:
(a) a benign chondroblastoma most commonly occurs in children under the age of 10
(b) a chondromyxoid fibroma most commonly involves the epiphysis
(c) calcification in the tumour is a feature of chondromyxoid fibroma
(d) sarcomatous change is more likely to occur in a chondroma of a flat bone
(e) a chondrosarcoma can arise in soft tissue

A9 Amyloidosis
(a) causes thickening of the small bowel wall
(b) occurs in 80% of patients with multiple myeloma
(c) causes endobronchial stenosis
(d) causes constrictive cardiomyopathy
(e) causes small kidneys

A10 An intrahepatic transonic lesion with an echogenic margin could be
(a) a haematoma
(b) a hydatid cyst
(c) a lymphoma deposit
(d) a tuberculoma
(e) an amoebic abscess

A11 The following features suggest malignancy in a lesion seen on mammogram:
(a) the lesion appearing larger on the radiograph than the clinical examination suggests

(b) increased vascularity
(c) enlargement of the lactiferous ducts
(d) displacement of trabeculae
(e) perifocal haziness

A12 Progressive massive fibrosis can occur in
(a) bagassosis
(b) barytosis
(c) silicosis
(d) coalworkers' pneumoconiosis
(e) stannosis

A13 When a meningioma is present
(a) hyperostosis occurs at the site of the lesion
(b) calcification is seen in 50% of cases on a plain radiograph
(c) enlargement of the foramen spinosum can be seen
(d) narrowing of the superior orbital fissure can occur
(e) lesions can be multiple in 10% of cases

A14 Causes of nasal bone erosion include
(a) sarcoidosis
(b) Wegener's granuloma
(c) bismuth poisoning
(d) cocaine addiction
(e) polyarteritis nodosa

A15 Fat embolism
(a) is confirmed by finding fat globules in centrifuged urine
(b) usually occurs less than 12 hours post trauma
(c) is associated with vitreous haemorrhages
(d) is associated with petechiae
(e) is seen in acute pancreatitis

A16 Gas within the biliary tree can be seen on the plain abdominal radiograph in
(a) mesenteric infarction
(b) patients who have had sphincterotomy of the lower end of the common bile duct
(c) gallstone ileus
(d) amoebic abscess
(e) choledochocoele

A17 In the Klippel–Feil syndrome
(a) multiple fused vertebral bodies are present
(b) there may be fusion of the posterior arches
(c) deafness occurs
(d) only the cervical vertebrae are involved
(e) Sprengel's deformity may occur

A18 Splenic calcification occurs in
(a) coeliac disease
(b) Gaucher's disease
(c) brucellosis
(d) sickle cell disease
(e) malaria

A19 Cone-shaped epiphyses in the phalanges can be seen
(a) after frostbite
(b) as a normal variant
(c) in cleidocranial dysostosis
(d) in osteogenesis imperfecta
(e) in sickle cell anaemia

A20 In Fallot's tetralogy
(a) a right-sided aorta occurs in 75% of patients
(b) the twelfth rib is often absent
(c) the majority have associated atrial septal defects
(d) there is an association with Turner's syndrome
(e) cyanosis does not occur at birth

A21 On computerised tomographic head scan a subdural haematoma
(a) can cause a hyperdense collection in the Sylvian fissure
(b) loses its crescentric configuration with time
(c) usually becomes isodense between 7 and 10 days after injury
(d) can be better demonstrated when isodense by the injection of contrast
(e) will be of low attenuation when longstanding

A22 Asbestos exposure causes
(a) an increased frequency of carcinoma of the bronchus
(b) bilateral pleural plaques
(c) an increased incidence of tuberculosis
(d) hypertrophic pulmonary osteoarthropathy in the majority
(e) few clinical signs even with radiographic changes of interstitial fibrosis

A23 In thyroid radioisotope scanning the following are correct
(a) a thyroid abscess will usually appear as an area of increased activity
(b) approximately 25% of the metastases of well differentiated carcinomas show uptake of ^{131}I
(c) medullary carcinomas usually take up ^{123}I
(d) a normal thyroid scan does not exclude carcinoma

(e) Hashimoto's thyroiditis usually gives diffusely increased activity

A24   On a barium examination of the small bowel
(a) giardiasis can be a cause of small nodular filling defects
(b) carcinoid tumours produce intraluminal filling defects
(c) short stenoses due to bands are demonstrated well on a 'follow-through' examination
(d) iregular filling defects in the terminal ileum may be caused by *Yersinia enterocolitica*
(e) thickened valvulae conniventes are seen in scleroderma

A25   In hypophosphatasia
(a) resolution of abnormalities seen on the radiograph occurs with vitamin D therapy
(b) metaphyseal fractures are common
(c) excess phosphoethanolamine is excreted in the urine
(d) the age of onset is related to severity of disease
(e) raised intracranial pressure occurs

A26   A sequestrated segment of lung
(a) most commonly occurs in the left lower lobe
(b) can present as a cavitating lesion on the chest radiograph
(c) has a blood supply from the pulmonary artery
(d) may be demonstrated on a bronchogram
(e) usually drains into the azygos system

A27   Causes of a dissecting aortic aneurysm include
(a) Marfan's syndrome
(b) Ehlers–Danlos syndrome
(c) heroin addiction
(d) pregnancy
(e) Turner's syndrome

A28   Calcification within soft tissues is seen in
(a) dermatomyositis
(b) Christian–Weber disease
(c) leprosy
(d) pseudohypoparathyroidism
(e) hypervitaminosis A

A29   Periosteal reactions are seen in children with
(a) juvenile chronic arthritis
(b) hypervitaminosis A
(c) sickle cell anaemia
(d) scurvy
(e) hypophosphatasia

A30 **In the colon**
 (a) the incidence of malignancy in tubular adenomas is low
 (b) polyps in the descending colon have a higher incidence of malignancy than those in the ascending colon
 (c) a polyp larger than 1 cm in diameter should be suspected of malignancy
 (d) the incidence of malignancy in familial polyposis is about 10%
 (e) juvenile polyps are more common in girls

A

Answers

A1
(a) **T** hypoplasia or absence of the medial third of the clavicle
(b) **F**
(c) **T** one or both clavicles may be partially or completely absent
(d) **T**
(e) **F**

A2
(a) **T**
(b) **T**
(c) **T**
(d) **F**
(e) **F**

A3
(a) **T** the Maisoneuve fracture
(b) **F** this occurs particularly in joggers. Ballet dancers tend to get stress fractures in the proximal tibia
(c) **F** occur with inversion injury
(d) **T**
(e) **T**

A4
(a) **F** idiopathic but definite familial incidence
(b) **T** also metacarpal, proximal and distal inter-phalangeal joints
(c) **T**
(d) **F** calcium pyrophosphate
(e) **T**

A5
(a) **T** if there is sufficient abdominal fat
(b) **T**
(c) **F**
(d) **F** metastases are most commonly from bron-chogenic carcinoma
(e) **F** the normal contours are maintained

A6
(a) **T** matrix stones

(b) **T**

(c) **T**

(d) **F**

(e) **T**

A7

(a) **F** usually about L5 with thickening of filum terminale

(b) **T** frequently but not invariably

(c) **T** about 20%

(d) **T**

(e) **T**

A8

(a) **F** second decade

(b) **F** metaphysis with extension into diaphysis

(c) **F**

(d) **T**

(e) **T**

A9

(a) **T**

(b) **F** in about 20%

(c) **T**

(d) **T**

(e) **F** kidneys are normal or enlarged in size

A10

(a) **T**

(b) **T**

(c) **T**

(d) **F** central calcification

(e) **T**

A11

(a) **F** appears smaller on radiograph

(b) **T** may be also seen in inflammatory conditions

(c) **T** due to intraduct tumour or distal destruction

(d) **F** trabeculae are destroyed, thickened or distorted in malignant disease

(e) **T** found in aggressive tumours. Also seen in inflammatory breast disease

A12

(a) **F**

(b) **F** extreme radio-opaque nodulation occurs without development of fibrosis

(c) **T**

(d) **T**

(e) **F**

A13

(a) **T**

(b)	**F**	15%
(c)	**T**	
(d)	**T**	
(e)	**F**	

A14

(a)	**T**	
(b)	**T**	
(c)	**F**	chromium oxide poisoning
(d)	**T**	
(e)	**F**	

A15

(a)	**T**	
(b)	**F**	two or three days
(c)	**F**	fat globules may be seen in retinal vessels
(d)	**T**	
(e)	**T**	

A16

(a)	**F**	
(b)	**T**	
(c)	**T**	
(d)	**T**	
(e)	**F**	

A17

(a)	**T**	
(b)	**T**	
(c)	**T**	30%
(d)	**F**	There is rarely also involvement of thoracic and lumbar areas
(e)	**T**	

A18

(a)	**F**	
(b)	**F**	
(c)	**T**	
(d)	**T**	
(e)	**F**	

A19

(a)	**T**	
(b)	**T**	
(c)	**T**	
(d)	**F**	
(e)	**T**	

A20

(a)	**F**	about one-third
(b)	**T**	
(c)	**F**	about 10% have ASD—Fallot's pentalogy

(d) **F**
(e) **F** a small number are cyanosed at birth

A21
(a) **F**
(b) **F**
(c) **F** usually two to four weeks before becoming isodense
(d) **T** contrast enhances the capsule
(e) **T**

A22
(a) **T**
(b) **T** usually diaphragmatic and pericardial
(c) **F**
(d) **F** very rare, even with mesothelioma
(e) **F** late inspiratory crackles correlate well with radiographic change

A23
(a) **F** usually appears as a cold area
(b) **F** 75% metastases take up ^{131}I in well differentiated carcinoma
(c) **F** rarely
(d) **T**
(e) **F** activity can vary from no activity to increased activity

A24
(a) **T**
(b) **T** usually in ileo caecal region
(c) **F** often missed and small bowel enema required for demonstration
(d) **T**
(e) **F** the valvulae conniventes are not usually thickened in the dilated segments

A25
(a) **F** vitamin D is contraindicated. There is no specific therapy
(b) **T**
(c) **T**
(d) **T** neonatal onset is lethal
(e) **T** due to craniostenosis. Initially wide cranial sutures may fuse prematurely

A26
(a) **T**
(b) **T**
(c) **F** separate branch from aorta
(d) **T**
(e) **F** into pulmonary veins

A27
- (a) **T**
- (b) **T**
- (c) **F**
- (d) **T**
- (e) **F**

A28
- (a) **T**
- (b) **T** subcutaneous nodules
- (c) **T** within nerves
- (d) **T** especially hands and feet
- (e) **F**

A29
- (a) **T**
- (b) **T**
- (c) **T** hand-foot syndrome
- (d) **T** most commonly occur in the lower limbs
- (e) **F**

A30
- (a) **T**
- (b) **T**
- (c) **T**
- (d) **F** 80% develop carcinoma
- (e) **F** boys

B

Questions

B1 The following are radiographic indications of fetal death:
(a) radiolucent blood vessels
(b) separation of cranial sutures
(c) elevation of pericranial fat
(d) position of extreme extension
(e) radiolucency of fetal bladder

B2 Patent ductus arteriosus
(a) commonly causes enlargement of the aortic knuckle
(b) can cause cardiac failure in infancy
(c) is associated with the rubella syndrome
(d) is not associated with subacute bacterial endocarditis
(e) can be therapeutically induced to close in the infant

B3 In miliary tuberculosis
(a) the Heaf test is usually positive
(b) there is fine nodularity throughout the lung fields on chest radiography
(c) mediastinal lymphadenopathy is a feature
(d) the diagnosis can sometimes be confirmed by examination of the fundi
(e) the radiological appearance improves within two weeks of onset of therapy

B4 In symptomatic stenosis of the internal carotid artery the following are recognised features
(a) transient episodes of deafness
(b) fibromuscular hypertrophy of the vessel
(c) the Foster Kennedy syndrome (ipsilateral optic atrophy and contralateral papilloedema)
(d) transient episodes of blindness
(e) previous oral contraceptive ingestion

B5 The use of glucagon is contraindicated in
(a) hypertension
(b) benign prostatic hypertrophy
(c) patients taking digitalis

(d) closed-angle glaucoma
(e) phaeochromocytoma

B6 Causes of rectal stricture include
(c) lymphogranuloma venereum
(b) schistosomiasis
(c) pelvic lipomatosis
(d) cervical carcinoma
(e) Stein–Leventhal syndrome

B7 Acromegaly
(a) produces expansion of the vertebral bodies
(b) produces widened joint spaces in the fingers
(c) is commonly due to a basophilic pituitary tumour
(d) is associated with bitemporal hemianopia
(e) is associated with a small liver

B8 In herpes simplex encephalitis
(a) preceding oro-labial lesions are seen
(b) on computerised tomographic brain scanning low density areas in both temporal lobes are typical
(c) on radioisotopic brain scanning bilateral areas of decreased activity occur
(d) brain biopsy is required for definitive diagnosis
(e) erythrocytosis of the cerebrospinal fluid indicates a poor prognosis

B9 On computerised tomographic examination of the abdomen
(a) abnormalities are seen in the spleen in about 90% of patients with histological proved lymphoma
(b) splenunculi can be identified
(c) congenital splenic cysts are commonly seen
(d) widespread areas of low density in the spleen may be produced by sickle cell disease
(e) low density areas may be seen in Morrison's pouch in splenic trauma

B10 On ultrasound examination of the liver
(a) focal hepatitis can cause an appearance indistinguishable from metastases
(b) pyogenic abscesses are commoner in the left lobe
(c) metastases from the urogenital tract can be echogenic
(d) fatty change results in uniform increased echogenicity
(e) established hydatid cysts have a characteristic appearance

B11 In tuberous sclerosis there is
(a) sclerosis of the distal phalanges
(b) an increased incidence of hamartoma of the kidney

(c)   an increased incidence of hepatoma
(d)   an increased incidence of cardiac rhabdomyoma
(e)   an increased incidence of cerebral glioma

B12   The following are associated
(a)   polyostotic fibrous dysplasia and precocious puberty
(b)   medullary carcinoma of the thyroid and phaeochromocytoma
(c)   Cushing's disease and squamous cell carcinoma of the bronchus
(d)   polycythaemia and medulloblastoma
(e)   hepatic adenoma and the contraceptive pill

B13   On pulmonary scintigraphy
(a)   the perfusion scan may be normal with a 'saddle' embolus
(b)   matching ventilation—perfusion defects can be seen in asthmatics
(c)   a repeat perfusion scan done after a week of therapy can show resolution of defects due to pulmonary emboli
(d)   a reduction in dose of radioisotope is required in perfusion scans done on patients with pulmonary hypertension
(e)   more than two views of the lung fields are required to exclude significant embolus

B14   A nephroblastoma
(a)   occurs in children under 5
(b)   is associated with horseshoe kidney
(c)   is bilateral in about 5% of cases
(d)   metastasises most commonly to bone
(e)   rarely calcifies

B15   Hepatic vein thrombosis
(a)   is associated with sickle cell anaemia
(b)   can occur following ingestion of senecio alkaloids
(c)   can be confirmed by technetium-99m colloid liver scan
(d)   usually presents with variceal bleeding
(e)   may be associated with intestinal infarction

B16   In Perthe's disease
(a)   the femoral head is displaced medially
(b)   changes in the metaphysis do not occur
(c)   concurrent changes in the other femoral head are very rare
(d)   intra-epiphyseal gas is seen
(e)   in most cases there is retardation of skeletal maturity

B17 The incidence of gastrointestinal malignancy is increased in
(a) Turcot's syndrome
(b) Peutz–Jeghers syndrome
(c) acanthosis nigricans
(d) erythema reticulatum
(e) Cronkhite–Canada syndrome

B18 Cystic fibrosis
(a) has an autosomal dominant inheritance
(b) is associated with gallstones
(c) is confirmed by a sweat test
(d) causes a highly echogenic pancreas on ultrasound
(e) produces diagnostic ultrasonic changes in the liver

B19 In acute head injury
(a) CT scanning is a reliable way of excluding fresh intracranial haemorrhage
(b) CSF otorrhoea is an indication for a horizontal beam lateral skull film
(c) rupture of the middle meningeal artery is commonly associated with overlying fracture
(d) immediate skull radiographs are mandatory
(e) management is affected by the demonstration of a linear vault fracture

B20 Chylothorax is associated with
(a) Whipple's disease
(b) Hodgkin's disease
(c) pulmonary lymphangiomyomatosis
(d) blunt chest trauma
(e) lymphangitis carcinomatosa

B21 Acute renal obstruction due to a stone can produce the following appearances on intravenous urogram
(a) absent psoas outline on the obstructed side
(b) filling defect in the bladder at the ureteric orifice
(c) a nephrogram of increasing density
(d) a scoliosis of the lumbar spine concave to the non-obstructed side
(e) peri-renal extravasation of contrast

B22 Increased splenic activity compared to the liver on a colloid radioisotope scan occurs in
(a) coeliac disease
(b) cryptogenic cirrhosis
(c) Budd–Chiari syndrome
(d) sickle cell anaemia
(e) renal failure

B23 **There is an association between pneumothorax and**
- (a) scleroderma
- (b) tuberculosis
- (c) aortic incompetence
- (d) mesothelioma
- (e) histiocytosis X

B24 **Pericardial calcification is caused by**
- (a) radiotherapy to the mediastinum
- (b) methysergide therapy
- (c) anticoagulant therapy
- (d) benign pericarditis
- (e) dermatomyositis

B25 **On renal ultrasound**
- (a) the kidney may appear normal in the presence of ureteric obstruction
- (b) distension of the bladder without outlet obstruction can cause a dilated pelvicalyceal system
- (c) parapelvic cysts can be indistinguishable from a hydronephrosis
- (d) focal scarring is not detectable
- (e) multicystic kidney can be indistinguishable from infantile polycystic kidney

B26 **The bronchial arteries**
- (a) are not visible on a chest radiograph in a normal patient
- (b) can be seen in Fallot's tetralogy
- (c) are seen on the chest radiograph when enlarged secondary to lung disease
- (d) usually arise from the descending aorta at T5 or T6 level
- (e) cause posterior rib notching when enlarged

B27 **The bony changes due to Sudeck's atrophy**
- (a) extend to the joint proximal to the site of injury
- (b) include erosions of the articular margins
- (c) are associated with overlying skin changes
- (d) may resolve spontaneously
- (e) are associated with calcification of small arteries

B28 **At arthrography**
- (a) of the knee, a discoid meniscus is more commonly seen on the medial side
- (b) of the knee, contrast medium does not usually enter the bursa surrounding the tendon of popliteus
- (c) of the ankle, contrast medium in the peroneal tendon sheath indicates a torn calcaneofibular ligament

(d) of the ankle, filling of the tendon sheath of flexor hallucis longus is abnormal

(e) of the shoulder joint, opacification of the subacromial bursa with contrast is due to a rotator cuff tear

B29 Early epiphyseal fusion occurs in
(a) adrenogenital syndrome
(b) homocystinuria
(c) phenylketonia
(d) Turner's syndrome
(e) Fanconi's syndrome

B30 When a computerised tomographic examination of the chest is performed
(a) in the lateral decubitus position the lowermost lung is in a state of relative respiratory apnoea
(b) most metastases are seen in the outer third of the lung fields
(c) cavitation in a pulmonary nodule is an indication of malignancy
(d) the mediastinal structures are well demonstrated in Cushing's disease
(e) a granuloma can be distinguished from a metastasis by the irregularity of its margins

B

Answers

B1
(a) **T**
(b) **F** overlap
(c) **T**
(d) **F** extreme flexion
(e) **F**

B2
(a) **T** 50% of cases. Not usually seen before the age of 10
(b) **T**
(c) **T**
(d) **F**
(e) **T** treated with indomethacin

B3
(a) **F**
(b) **T**
(c) **F**
(d) **T** choroidal tubercles are diagnostic
(e) **F** radiological changes take a long time to improve and may even look worse

B4
(a) **F**
(b) **T**
(c) **F** occurs in frontal lobe tumours
(d) **T**
(e) **F**

B5
(a) **F**
(b) **F**
(c) **F**
(d) **F**
(e) **T**

B6
(a) **T**
(b) **T**
(c) **F**
(d) **T**
(e) **F**

B7
- (a) **T** wider in the coronal plane and deeper than usual
- (b) **T** due to thickening of the articular cartilage
- (c) **F** eosinophilic or mixed cell tumours
- (d) **T**
- (e) **F** hypertrophy of the liver

B8
- (a) **F**
- (b) **T**
- (c) **F** increased activity
- (d) **T**
- (e) **T**

B9
- (a) **F** about 50%
- (b) **F**
- (c) **F** they are very rare
- (d) **T**
- (e) **F** fresh blood is of high density

B10
- (a) **T** multiple anechoic lesions
- (b) **F**
- (c) **T** also from gut and occasionally bronchus and breast
- (d) **T**
- (e) **T** when no daughter cysts are present the appearance is that of a simple cyst

B11
- (a) **T**
- (b) **T**
- (c) **F**
- (d) **T**
- (e) **T**

B12
- (a) **T** Albright's syndrome
- (b) **T**
- (c) **F** oat cell carcinoma of bronchus
- (d) **F**
- (e) **T**

B13
- (a) **T** extremely rare
- (b) **T**
- (c) **T** partial resolution is often seen
- (d) **F** the dose of radioisotope is the same, but fewer particles are desirable
- (e) **T**

B14
- (a) **T**
- (b) **T** also other congenital malformation, e.g. hemihypertrophy and aniridia
- (c) **T**
- (d) **F** lung
- (e) **T**

B15
- (a) **T**
- (b) **T** bush teas are the commonest cause
- (c) **T** the characteristic scan is not always obtained
- (d) **F** abdominal pain and ascites
- (e) **T** due to retrograde thrombus

B16
- (a) **F** the femoral head is displaced laterally
- (b) **F** metaphyseal rarefaction is not uncommon
- (c) **T** bilateral changes occur but at different times
- (d) **T** seen in the radiographic frog leg position
- (e) **T** skeletal maturity may be delayed by six months to three years

B17
- (a) **F** recessive transmitted disorder with colonic adenomas and CNS tumours
- (b) **T**
- (c) **T**
- (d) **F**
- (e) **T** syndrome of alopecia, hyperpigmentation, diarrhoea and polyps throughout the bowel

B18
- (a) **F** autosomal recessive with variable penetrance
- (b) **T**
- (c) **T**
- (d) **T**
- (e) **F** increased heterogeneous echogenicity which is also seen in cirrhosis

B19
- (a) **T**
- (b) **T** to show air/fluid level
- (c) **T**
- (d) **F**
- (e) **F**

B20
- (a) **F**
- (b) **T**
- (c) **T**
- (d) **T**
- (e) **F**

B21
(a) **T**
(b) **T** due to oedema surrounding impacted stone
(c) **T**
(d) **F** concavity towards the obstructed side
(e) **T**

B22
(a) **F**
(b) **T**
(c) **T**
(d) **F**
(e) **F**

B23
(a) **T**
(b) **T** bronchopleural fistula from cavitating lesion
(c) **T** Marfan's syndrome
(d) **F**
(e) **T** 'Honeycomb' lung

B24
(a) **T**
(b) **T**
(c) **T** secondary to haematoma
(d) **T**
(e) **F**

B25
(a) **T**
(b) **T**
(c) **T**
(d) **F**
(e) **T**

B26
(a) **T**
(b) **T** dilate in response to hypoxia
(c) **F** arteriography required to demonstrate them
(d) **T** although they may arise from internal mammary or brachiocephalic arteries
(e) **F**

B27
(a) **F** confined to bones distal to injury
(b) **F**
(c) **T** skin is smooth, shiny and swollen
(d) **T**
(e) **F**

B28
(a) **F** lateral
(b) **F**

(c)   **T**

(d)   **F**   can occur in normal ankles

(e)   **T**

B29

(a)   **T**

(b)   **T**

(c)   **F**

(d)   **F**

(e)   **F**

B30

(a)   **F**   uppermost lung

(b)   **T**

(c)   **F**

(d)   **T**   due to the abnormal quantity of fat

(e)   **F**   some metastases, e.g. choriocarcinoma, have
irregular margins

C

Questions

C1 In achondroplasia
(a) there is a decrease in the interpedicular distance from L1 to L5
(b) the first lumbar vertebra is 'bullet' shaped
(c) the epiphyses are frequently small
(d) the foramen magnum is small
(e) the paranasal sinuses are underdeveloped

C2 In coeliac disease
(a) there is flattening of the valvulae conniventes on a small bowel meal in 10% of patients
(b) lymphoma is a complication
(c) transient intussusception may be seen during a small bowel examination
(d) ulcers may develop in the small bowel
(e) there is an association with histocompatibility antigen HLA-B8

C3 Syringomyelia
(a) produces neurological signs in upper and lower limbs
(b) commonly involves the dorsal columns
(c) is associated with a scoliosis
(d) is commonly associated with Arnold–Chiari malformation
(e) presents in children under 10 years of age

C4 On a lymphangiogram
(a) there can be a 'soap bubble' appearance of the lymph nodes in metastatic seminoma
(b) enlarged lymph nodes can be seen in lymphatic leukaemia
(c) the nodes involved in Hodgkin's disease differ in appearance from lymphosarcoma
(d) tuberculous lymphadenitis can simulate metastatic disease
(e) contrast medium will remain in pathological lymph nodes for only two months

C5 Bronchial carcinoid
(a) can present as a rounded peripheral lesion on chest radiograph
(b) rarely causes haemoptysis

(c) is usually associated with the carcinoid syndrome
(d) is locally invasive
(e) is commoner in the lower lobe

C6 In renal artery stenosis
(a) a delayed nephrogram is seen on the affected side
(b) a small kidney is typical
(c) filling defects in the ureter on intravenous urogram are seen
(d) a dense nephrogram is seen on the contralateral side
(e) Takayasu disease can be the cause

C7 Gynaecomastia is seen in association with
(a) carcinoma of the bronchus
(b) carcinoma of the thyroid
(c) cryptogenic fibrosing alveolitis
(d) Klinefelter's syndrome
(e) amphetamine therapy

C8 The following can cause soft tissue calcification on a plain radiograph of the pelvis
(a) *Schistosoma mansoni* infection
(b) serous cystadenocarcinoma of ovary
(c) papilloma of bladder
(d) endometriosis
(e) colloid carcinoma of the colon

C9 When a pericardial effusion is present
(a) at least 150 ml of fluid must have accumulated before there is a change in the cardiac outline on the chest radiograph
(b) it is best seen behind the left atrium on real time ultrasound
(c) a swinging motion of the heart is seen on real time ultrasound
(d) pulsus paradoxus is associated with cardiac tamponade
(e) the jugular venous pressure is elevated if tamponade is present

C10 An elevated paralysed hemi-diaphragm can be seen in
(a) herpes zoster
(b) Chilaiditi syndrome
(c) eventration
(d) perinephric abscess
(e) systemic lupus erythematosis

C11 Urethral strictures
(a) resulting from infection usually involve the membranous region

(b) predispose to renal calculi
(c) in the posterior urethra are best demonstrated by retrograde urethrography
(d) occur with Peyronie's disease
(e) following pelvic trauma usually involve the anterior urethra

C12 Increased focal activity on a technetium-99m brain scan could be due to
(a) a week-old cerebral infarct
(b) a scalp haematoma
(c) a leptomeningeal cyst
(d) a pituitary tumour
(e) a syphilitic gumma

C13 The following are correct:
(a) spinal damage occurs in association with about 10% of calcaneal crush injuries
(b) adduction of the proximal fragment of a femoral shaft fracture suggests there may be a posterior hip dislocation
(c) a nerve palsy resulting from a fracture of the humeral shaft most commonly involves the radial nerve
(d) about 5% of patients with a spinal fracture have a second fracture at another level
(e) resorption of the medial end of the clavicle can occur following fracture

C14 Looser's zones
(a) commonly occur in the femoral neck
(b) are associated with elevated serum alkaline phosphatase
(c) are seen in biliary atresia
(d) are seen in Cushing's syndrome
(e) are a complication of anti-convulsant therapy

C15 In the colon
(a) Peutz–Jeghers polyps do not become malignant
(b) a villous adenoma can be associated with hypocalcaemia
(c) there is an increased incidence of malignancy with polyps with bases larger than 2 cm in diameter
(d) a solitary polyp can disappear spontaneously
(e) metaplastic rectal polyps are not premalignant

C16 A peripheral neuropathy may occur in
(a) infectious mononucleosis
(b) polyarteritis nodosa
(c) polyvinyl chloride poisoning

(d) cystic fibrosis
(e) amyloidosis

C17 When computerised tomographic examination of the abdomen is performed in a patient with pancreatitis
(a) marked irregularity of the pancreatic duct is highly suggestive of chronic pancreatitis
(b) a focal mass in the body of the pancreas is highly suggestive of carcinoma
(c) extra-pancreatic fluid collections are nearly always present in acute pancreatitis
(d) pancreatic calcification can be shown even if plain radiographs appear normal
(e) there is loss of the tissue plane between pancreas and aorta

C18 Carpal fusion is seen in
(a) juvenile chronic arthritis
(b) Ellis–van Creveld syndrome
(c) tuberculosis
(d) reticulo-histiocytosis
(e) hyperparathyroidism

C19 The heart size
(a) is usually normal in isolated pulmonary stenosis
(b) can be normal in a patient with critical mitral stenosis
(c) is often normal in ventriculo-septal defects
(d) is normal in Ebstein's anomaly
(e) can be normal in Fallot's tetralogy

C20 In cryptogenic fibrosing alveolitis
(a) a gallium-67 scan will define the extent of the fibrosis
(b) if basal crackles are present on auscultation radiographic changes will be seen
(c) histological confirmation is readily acquired with a transbronchial biopsy
(d) finger clubbing is often present
(e) there is an increased incidence of bronchogenic carcinoma

C21 On renal ultrasound examination the cortical echo pattern is increased compared to adjacent liver/spleen echo pattern in
(a) diabetes
(b) renal transplant rejection
(c) lymphoma
(d) chronic glomerulonephritis
(e) sarcoidosis

C22 Meckel's diverticula
(a) occur in about 5% of the population
(b) sometimes contain calculi
(c) are rarely demonstrated on a small bowel meal
(d) will usually be demonstrated by a technetium-99m colloid scan
(e) are associated with accessory splenunculi

C23 Suprarenal calcification can occur in
(a) phaeochromocytoma
(b) Wolman's disease
(c) idiopathic hypercalcaemic syndrome
(d) Conn's syndrome
(e) histoplasmosis

C24 Oligaemia of one lung field is seen in
(a) primary pulmonary hypertension
(b) McLeod's syndrome
(c) Fallot's tetralogy
(d) pulmonary embolism without infarction
(e) bronchogenic carcinoma

C25 The absence of gas on an abdominal radiograph is suggestive of
(a) proximal small bowel obstruction
(b) psoas abscess
(c) chest infection
(d) mid-gut volvulus
(e) acute pancreatitis

C26 In toxoplasmosis
(a) neonatal congenital disease is usually mild
(b) calcification of the basal ganglia can be seen
(c) antimicrobial therapy is not always necessary in adults
(d) diagnosis is made by examination of the blood for parasites
(e) in infancy only a few cases have choroidoretinitis

C27 Nasopharyngeal angiofibromas
(a) usually present with epistaxis
(b) are more common in females
(c) are often demonstrated on angiography as a dense blush
(d) erode the posterior wall of the maxillary antrum
(e) usually have blood supply from the internal carotid arteries

C28 On an abdominal radiograph calcification may be seen in the bladder wall in
(a) tuberculous cystitis
(b) malacoplakia

(c) schistosomiasis
(d) cyclophosphamide cystitis
(e) diabetes mellitus

C29 Generalised cranial hyperostosis can be seen in
(a) osteopetrosis
(b) dystrophia myotonica
(c) phenobarbitone therapy
(d) hypothyroidism
(e) Engelmann's disease

C30 'Eggshell' calcification of enlarged hilar lymph nodes is seen in
(a) primary tuberculosis
(b) untreated lymphoma
(c) sarcoidosis
(d) asbestosis
(e) silicosis

C

Answers

C1
- (a) **T**
- (b) **T**
- (c) **F** epiphyses are normal
- (d) **T** hydrocephalus can occur
- (e) **F**

C2
- (a) **F** about 50% of patients
- (b) **T**
- (c) **T**
- (d) **T**
- (e) **T**

C3
- (a) **T**
- (b) **T**
- (c) **F**
- (d) **T**
- (e) **F** 20 to 40 years

C4
- (a) **T**
- (b) **T**
- (c) **F** the reticuloses all have similar appearances
- (d) **T**
- (e) **F** remains in nodes for at least six months

C5
- (a) **T**
- (b) **F** is highly vascular and recurrent haemoptyses are common
- (c) **F** rarely seen unless there are metastases
- (d) **T** invades locally with spread to mediastinal lymph nodes
- (e) **T**

C6
- (a) **T**
- (b) **T**
- (c) **T** due to impression by collateral vessels
- (d) **F**
- (e) **T**

C7
(a) **T**
(b) **F**
(c) **T**
(d) **T**
(e) **T**

C8
(a) **F** *Schistosoma japonicum* or *haematobium*
(b) **T**
(c) **T** encrustation of calcium salts
(d) **F**
(e) **T**

C9
(a) **T**
(b) **F** the pericardium is absent at this site
(c) **T** seen with moderate to large effusions
(d) **T**
(e) **T**

C10
(a) **T**
(b) **F** interposition of hepatic flexure between diaphragm and liver
(c) **F**
(d) **T**
(e) **F**

C11
(a) **F** bulbous urethra
(b) **T**
(c) **F** this does not always fill the posterior urethra adequately and antegrade urethrography should be done
(d) **F**
(e) **F** posterior urethra

C12
(a) **T**
(b) **T**
(c) **F**
(d) **T**
(e) **T**

C13
(a) **T**
(b) **T**
(c) **T**
(d) **T**
(e) **F** lateral end of clavicle

C14
(a) **T** medial cortex
(b) **T**
(c) **T** because of associated osteomalacia
(d) **F** osteoporosis occurs
(e) **T** phenytoin therapy

C15
(a) **T**
(b) **F** hypokalaemia
(c) **T**
(d) **T** by torsion and infarction of the pedicle
(e) **T**

C16
(a) **T**
(b) **T**
(c) **F**
(d) **F**
(e) **T**

C17
(a) **T**
(b) **T**
(c) **F** occurs in less than 20% in the lesser sac and anterior para-renal space
(d) **T**
(e) **T**

C18
(a) **T** usually symmetrical
(b) **T**
(c) **T**
(d) **F**
(e) **F**

C19
(a) **T** even in severe stenosis
(b) **T** in 10% of patients
(c) **T**
(d) **F**
(e) **T**

C20
(a) **F** the amount of uptake depends on cellular activity and diminishes as fibrosis becomes more extensive
(b) **F** the chest radiograph may be normal with widespread crackles
(c) **F** open lung biopsy is often required
(d) **T**
(e) **T** tenfold increase

C21

(a) **T**
(b) **T**
(c) **F**
(d) **T**
(e) **T**

C22

(a) **F** 0.01% of the population
(b) **T**
(c) **T** small bowel enema more likely to show it
(d) **F** pertechnetate scan, or labelled red cell scan if bleeding
(e) **T**

C23

(a) **T**
(b) **T** stippled calcification of enlarged adrenals
(c) **F**
(d) **T** uncommon. Thought to be due to haemorrhage into an adenoma
(e) **T**

C24

(a) **F** both lung fields have reduced vascularity
(b) **T** obstructive emphysema with oligaemic lung
(c) **T** usually left lung is less vascular
(d) **T** a large embolus can obstruct the pulmonary artery
(e) **T**

C25

(a) **T**
(b) **F**
(c) **F**
(d) **F**
(e) **T**

C26

(a) **F** severe, most die in infancy
(b) **T** but unusual, more often grey/white junction
(c) **T** most immunologically normal patients do not require treatment unless symptoms are severe
(d) **F** complement fixation
(e) **F** all have choroidoretinitis

C27

(a) **T**
(b) **F**
(c) **T** very vascular
(d) **F** cause anterior bowing, not erosion
(e) **F** external carotid

C28
- (a) **T** uncommon
- (b) **F**
- (c) **T**
- (d) **T**
- (e) **F**

C29
- (a) **T**
- (b) **T**
- (c) **F** phenytoin
- (d) **F**
- (e) **T**

C30
- (a) **F**
- (b) **F** peripheral calcification can occur after treatment
- (c) **T**
- (d) **F**
- (e) **T**

D

Questions

D1 Multiple Wormian bones can be seen in
(a) neonatal hypothyroidism
(b) Down's syndrome
(c) fibrous dysplasia
(d) progeria
(e) normal babies

D2 Hypertrophic pulmonary osteoarthropathy occurs with
(a) fibrosing alveolitis
(b) pleural fibroma
(c) squamous carcinoma of the bronchus
(d) myeloma deposits in ribs
(e) pulmonary metastases of osteogenic sarcoma

D3 'Thumb-printing' of the colon on a barium enema can be seen in
(a) diverticular disease
(b) acute intussusception
(c) ischaemic colitis
(d) Crohn's disease
(e) endometriosis

D4 Causes of a posterior soft tissue nasopharyngeal mass include
(a) plasmacytoma
(b) choanal atresia
(c) Thornwaldt's cyst
(d) aneurysm of the carotid artery
(e) chordoma

D5 Pulmonary hamartomas
(a) are usually seen in children
(b) have a female predominance
(c) can have satellite lesions
(d) always have calcification demonstrable on CT examination
(e) are supplied by the bronchial arteries

D6 The following are manifestations of neurofibromatosis:
(a) sclerosis of the orbital walls

(b) osteomalacia
(c) hypertrophy of a limb
(d) renal artery aneurysms
(e) optic nerve glioma

D7 Frontal mucocoeles
(a) cause displacement of the supraorbital ridge
(b) can present with unilateral exophthalmos
(c) cause surrounding sclerosis
(d) are rare compared to maxillary antral mucocoeles
(e) can occur with lacrimal gland neoplasms

D8 Osteonecrosis
(a) can occur in the shafts of bones after renal transplantation
(b) often involves bones on both sides of a joint
(c) in dysbaric disorders is commonly seen in the head of the femur
(d) will produce areas of increased activity on isotope bone scanning before changes are seen on a radiograph
(e) can simulate osteosarcoma on radiographs

D9 Renal calculi
(a) composed of xanthine are radiolucent
(b) occur in patients with cystinosis
(c) composed of uric acid occur as a familial disease in Scandinavians
(d) are more common in duplex kidneys
(e) composed of uric acid can be associated with inflammatory bowel disease

D10 In the spine
(a) neurofibromas are indistinguishable from meningiomas on myelography
(b) ependymomas are commonly found in the cervical region
(c) a lateral thoracic meningocoele usually presents with paraparesis
(d) gliomas usually occur in the thoracic region
(e) extradural cysts present in middle age

D11 Duodenal ulceration
(a) occurs with increased frequency in patients with chronic pancreatitis
(b) is more common in patients with blood group A
(c) is associated with polycythaemia
(d) occurs after severe burns
(e) is seen with increased frequency in patients with hyperparathyroidism

D12 Pathological fractures
(a) are commonly transverse in long bones
(b) in Paget's disease commonly occur in the shaft of the femur
(c) commonly occur in areas of chronic osteomyelitis
(d) occur in the subtrochanteric region of the femoral shaft
(e) occur as separation of the proximal femoral epiphysis in children with renal osteodystrophy

D13 In the knee joint
(a) avulsion of the anterior tibial spine commonly occurs as a solitary injury
(b) avulsion of the anterior tibial spine involves the origin of the posterior cruciate ligament
(c) ruptures of the quadriceps tendon are associated with changes on the lateral radiographs
(d) chronic subluxation of the patella is associated with a prominent lateral femoral condyle
(e) dislocation is associated with arterial damage

D14 When the abdomen has been exposed to radiation of therapeutic dosage
(a) the jejunum is damaged more commonly than the ileum
(b) a vasculitis is produced in the bowel wall
(c) stenoses in the bowel can occur
(d) the mucosa atrophies
(e) symptoms may develop after many years

D15 Atlanto-axial dislocation has been described in
(a) systemic lupus erythematosis
(b) progeria
(c) ankylosing spondylitis
(d) spondylo-epiphyseal dysplasia congenita
(e) tuberculosis

D16 In splenic rupture
(a) arteriography is contraindicated
(b) the left hemi-diaphragm is typically elevated
(c) ultrasound can demonstrate subcapsular haematomas
(d) infectious mononucleosis is a predisposing cause
(e) myelosclerosis is a predisposing cause

D17 In sarcoidosis
(a) there may be changes on the chest radiograph in an asymptomatic patient
(b) diabetes mellitus is a recognised complication
(c) hypercalcaemia always occurs in the acute disease
(d) the tuberculin reaction is often positive
(e) cardiac involvement may manifest as arrythmias

D18 In pulmonary embolism
- (a) the chest radiograph can be normal
- (b) mismatches in the ventilation-perfusion scan confirm the diagnosis
- (c) a negative lower limb venogram indicates a diagnosis other than pulmonary embolism
- (d) there can be small bilateral pleural effusions
- (e) localised oligaemia is sometimes seen on the chest radiograph

D19 In infantile cortical hyperostosis
- (a) the child is pyrexial
- (b) there can be associated pleural effusions
- (c) there is characteristically overlying soft tissue swelling
- (d) the average age of onset is six months
- (e) there is always complete resolution of the lesions

D20 With left atrial myxoma
- (a) pyrexia may be the presenting feature
- (b) calcification is sometimes seen on the plain chest radiograph
- (c) arterial emboli occur
- (d) there is an association with tuberous sclerosis
- (e) multiple tumours are rare

D21 Soft tissue calcification can be seen around the hip joint on a plain radiograph in
- (a) poliomyelitis
- (b) tumoral calcinosis
- (c) melorheostosis
- (d) polyostotic fibrous dysplasia
- (e) *Trichinella spiralis* infection

D22 Bilateral enlarged kidneys can be seen in
- (a) diabetes mellitus
- (b) acute tubular necrosis
- (c) acromegaly
- (d) Cushing's syndrome
- (e) multiple myeloma

D23 Coarse apical fibrosis on the chest radiograph is seen in
- (a) histoplasmosis
- (b) ankylosing spondylitis
- (c) phenacetin poisoning
- (d) psoriasis
- (e) severe kyphoscoliosis

D24 In ultrasound examination of the neck
- (a) a central, transonic, well-defined lesion could represent a branchial cleft cyst

(b) thyroid adenomas often have a transonic margin
(c) high level echoes can be seen with follicular carcinoma of the thyroid
(d) the more echogenic nodules seen in the thyroid the greater the likelihood that the lesion is benign
(e) normal parathyroid glands are usually less than 5 mm in diameter

D25 Steatorrhoea occurs in
(a) Whipple's disease
(b) gluten sensitivity
(c) giardiasis
(d) Addison's disease
(e) Peutz–Jeghers syndrome

D26 The following are features of the fetal alcohol syndrome:
(a) hypoplasia of the little finger
(b) hydrocephaly
(c) mild facial hypoplasia
(d) ventricular septal defect
(e) tender distal phalanges

D27 In acute pancreatitis
(a) the left psoas shadow may be absent on the abdominal radiograph
(b) pleural effusions are more common on the right
(c) the ultrasonic appearance of the pancreas can be normal in association with a very high serum amylase
(d) elevation of the serum calcium level is an indication of significant fat necrosis
(e) there is an association with carcinoma of the pancreas

D28 Loss of lamina dura of the teeth can occur in
(a) Paget's disease
(b) osteogenesis imperfecta
(c) histiocytosis X
(d) hypophosphatasia
(e) Cushing's syndrome

D29 In patients with renal lipoangiomata
(a) epileptic fits occur
(b) attacks of abdominal pain occur
(c) the renal angiogram is normal
(d) associated bone changes occur
(e) associated rhabdomyoma of the heart occurs

D30 A mass in the right anterior cardiophrenic angle could be
- (a) a hernia through foramen of Bochdalek
- (b) a neuroenteric cyst
- (c) spring water cyst
- (d) thymic cyst
- (e) secondary to steroid therapy

D

Answers

D1
(a) T
(b) T
(c) F
(d) T   premature aging syndrome
(e) T

D2
(a) T
(b) T
(c) T
(d) F
(e) T

D3
(a) F
(b) F
(c) T
(d) T
(e) T

D4
(a) T
(b) F
(c) T   notocord remnant
(d) T
(e) T

D5
(a) F   usually present in middle age
(b) F
(c) F
(d) F   70% do not calcify
(e) T

D6
(a) F   ossification of the sphenoid and posterior walls of the orbit may be defective
(b) T
(c) T
(d) T   occlusive arterial disease occurs, especially involving the renal arteries
(e) T

D7
(a) **T**
(b) **T**
(c) **T**
(d) **F**
(e) **T**

D8
(a) **T**
(b) **F**
(c) **T**
(d) **T**
(e) **T** history and biopsy should differentiate

D9
(a) **T**
(b) **F** cystinuria
(c) **F** occurs in east Mediterranean countries
(d) **T**
(e) **T**

D10
(a) **T**
(b) **F** sacral
(c) **F** asymptomatic
(d) **F** anywhere
(e) **F** second decade

D11
(a) **T**
(b) **F** group O
(c) **T**
(d) **T**
(e) **T**

D12
(a) **T**
(b) **T**
(c) **F** superimposed squamous cell carcinoma should be suspected
(d) **T**
(e) **T** occur in the proximal femoral and distal radial epiphyses

D13
(a) **T**
(b) **F** this is the origin of the anterior cruciate ligament
(c) **T** indentation is seen with soft tissue swelling proximal to the patella
(d) **F** this is associated with low lateral femoral condyle
(e) **T**

D14
- (a) F
- (b) T
- (c) T
- (d) T
- (e) T

D15
- (a) F
- (b) F
- (c) T
- (d) T
- (e) T   due to softening of ligaments from adjacent infection

D16
- (a) F
- (b) F
- (c) T
- (d) T
- (e) T

D17
- (a) T
- (b) F   diabetes insipidus
- (c) F   persistent hypercalcaemia can be seen in chronic disease
- (d) F
- (e) T

D18
- (a) T
- (b) T   provided that there are no other changes in the lung fields to account for them
- (c) F
- (d) T
- (e) T

D19
- (a) T
- (b) T
- (c) T
- (d) F   about nine weeks
- (e) F   cross union of paired bones is a known complication

D20
- (a) T
- (b) T
- (c) T
- (d) F   rhabdomyosarcomas seen in tuberous sclerosis
- (e) T

D21

(a) **T**

(b) **T**

(c) **T**

(d) **F**

(e) **F** too small to be seen on radiograph

D22

(a) **T**

(b) **T**

(c) **T**

(d) **F**

(e) **T**

D23

(a) **F** healing is not usually accompanied by fibrosis

(b) **T**

(c) **F**

(d) **F**

(e) **T**

D24

(a) **F** always lie laterally in the neck

(b) **T**

(d) **F** papillary carcinoma

(d) **T**

(e) **T**

D25

(a) **T**

(b) **T**

(c) **T**

(d) **T**

(e) **F**

D26

(a) **T** the little finger may be completely absent

(b) **F** microcephaly

(c) **T**

(d) **T**

(e) **T**

D27

(a) **T** however, this is a non-specific sign

(b) **F** more common on the left

(c) **T** an apparently normal pancreas does not exclude the diagnosis

(d) **F** fat necrosis causes a fall in the serum calcium

(e) **T**

D28

(a) **T**

- (b) **F**
- (c) **T**
- (d) **T**
- (e) **T**

D29
- (a) **T** associated with tuberous sclerosis in which epileptic fits are characteristic
- (b) **T** tumour may become necrotic or haemorrhagic
- (c) **F** there are abnormal dilated vessels and vascular lakes
- (d) **T**
- (e) **T**

D30
- (a) **F** Morgagni hernia
- (b) **F**
- (c) **T**
- (d) **T**
- (e) **T** due to fat deposition

E

Questions

E1 In extrinsic allergic alveolitis
(a) the patient may have a normal chest radiograph
(b) during the acute phase upper zone changes predominate
(c) hilar lymph node enlargement is frequently seen
(d) pleural effusions are common
(e) there is an eosinophilia in the acute stage

E2 Calcification of the ascending aorta occurs in
(a) Marfan's syndrome
(b) Reiter's syndrome
(c) aneurysms of sinus of Valsalva
(d) Takayasu's disease
(e) asbestosis

E3 Platybasia may be seen in
(a) osteogenesis imperfecta
(b) osteomalacia
(c) association with hypertelorism
(d) Engelmann's disease
(e) Cleidocranial dysostosis

E4 Adult polycystic renal disease is associated with
(a) splenic cysts
(b) portal hypertension
(c) arteriovenous malformation in lungs
(d) subarachnoid haemorrhage
(e) urinary stones

E5 Wolman's disease
(a) is a mucopolysaccharidosis
(b) is a cause of splenomegaly
(c) causes death in the second decade
(d) has a diagnostic appearance on the abdominal radiograph
(e) causes diarrhoea

E6 In sickle cell anaemia
(a) increased activity may be seen in the spleen on radioisotopic bone scanning
(b) a 'hair-on-end' appearance of the skull vault commonly develops

(c) florid periosteal reactions can be seen in infancy
(d) bone infarcts occur in tubular bones of the hands in children
(e) cholesterol gallstones are a common complication

E7 On computerised tomographic examination of the abdomen
(a) an area of high density around the aorta can be due to a fresh haematoma
(b) calcification may be seen in retroperitoneal fibrosis
(c) after radiotherapy for Hodgkin's disease lymph nodes increase in size
(d) lymph nodes involved in testicular cancer may show areas of low density
(e) involved nodes in Hodgkin's lymphoma may be of normal size

E8 The incidence of gallstones is increased in
(a) diabetes mellitus
(b) ischaemic heart disease
(c) pregnancy
(d) myelofibrosis
(e) thalassaemia

E9 In giant cell arteritis
(a) most patients present with temporal headache
(b) claudication of the jaw occurs
(c) occasionally the presenting symptom is bilateral visual loss
(d) shoulder pain is a recognised feature
(e) the plasma viscosity is normal

E10 In MacLeod's syndrome
(a) there is air trapping on the affected side
(b) the pulmonary perfusion radioisotope scan is normal
(c) there are characteristic changes on bronchography
(d) lobar involvement is frequent
(e) there is compensatory enlargement of the bronchial arteries in the affected lung

E11 An enlarged left atrium can be associated with
(a) splinter haemorrhages
(b) raised plasma viscosity
(c) a low rumbling diastolic murmur
(d) recurrent pulmonary emboli
(e) hypertrophic obstructive cardiomyopathy

E12 Diametaphyseal infarction of bone occurs in
(a) Gaucher's disease
(b) polyarteritis nodosa

- (c) thalassaemia
- (d) alcoholism
- (e) steroid therapy

E13 **A diffuse reduction in activity throughout the liver on a technetium-99m colloid scan can be seen in**
- (a) lymphoma
- (b) portal vein thrombosis
- (c) myelosclerosis
- (d) amoebic abcess
- (e) Budd–Chiari syndrome

E14 **An aneurysmal bone cyst**
- (a) is commonly seen after closure of the epiphyses
- (b) can be seen in any bone
- (c) can disrupt the cortex of the affected bone
- (d) is slow growing
- (e) can contain flecks of calcium

E15 **In the hand**
- (a) erosive changes in psoriasis commonly involve the distal interphalangeal joints
- (b) it is unusual to see radiographic bony changes during a first attack of gout
- (c) the erosive changes in gout are para-articular
- (d) the metacarpo-phalangeal joints are affected in haemochromatosis
- (e) erosive osteoarthritic changes are usually first seen in the proximal interphalangeal joints

E16 **On a barium meal examination widening of the duodenal loop suggests a diagnosis of**
- (a) pancreatic pseudocyst
- (b) choledochal cyst
- (c) Caroli's disease
- (d) acute aortic aneurysm
- (e) Budd–Chiari syndrome

E17 **The following are correct:**
- (a) a right-sided aortic arch is not usually associated with congenital cardiac defects
- (b) atrial septal defects are commoner in females
- (c) a ventricular septal defect can be associated with plethora of the right lung only
- (d) a large aortic arch is seen on the chest radiograph of infants with patent duct arteriosus
- (e) calcification in the aortic valve is indicative of significant stenosis

E18 **Intervertebral disc calcification occurs in**
- (a) ankylosing spondylitis

(b) homocystinuria
(c) hypervitaminosis D
(d) neurofibromatosis
(e) gout

E19 In a patient with a hypernephroma
(a) not infrequently the first symptoms arise from bony metastases
(b) calcification may be seen on an abdominal radiograph
(c) lactic dehydrogenase activity in the urine is normal
(d) polycythaemia can be a presenting feature
(e) a hypernephroma may be present in the other kidney

E20 In colitis cystica profunda
(a) males are more often affected than females
(b) on a barium enema the appearance is indistinguishable from rectal carcinoma
(c) hypokalemia can occur
(d) rectal strictures can occur
(e) the whole colon can be involved

E21 In blunt chest trauma
(a) the most commonly fractured ribs are the fourth to the ninth
(b) the chest radiograph can be normal with a ruptured diaphragm
(c) the radiographs can be normal with a bronchial tear
(d) an aortic tear usually begins in the ascending aorta
(e) pneumoperitoneum can occur without a pneumothorax

E22 On ultrasound examination of the pelvis
(a) a solid adnexal mass and ascites indicate malignant disease
(b) enlargement of uterine fibroid before the menopause suggests malignant degeneration
(c) septa can be shown in an ovarian mass which appears homogeneous on a CT scan
(d) fixity of a largely solid adnexal mass indicates malignancy
(e) cysts of the ovary are associated with hydatidiform moles

E23 In trisomy 18 syndrome
(a) hypoplastic ribs are typical
(b) the acetabular roof is flat
(c) the first metacarpal is short

(d) there is a lumbar kyphoscoliosis
(e) 'rocker bottom' feet are characteristic

E24   In coronary artery disease
(a) injection of thallium-201 immediately after exercise will demonstrate ischaemic areas in the myocardium
(b) an absent area of activity 20 minutes after injection of thallium-201 indicates infarction
(c) a left ventricular aneurysm is commonly seen on plain radiography of the chest
(d) the ejection fraction of the left ventricle can be calculated on a MUGA isotope scan
(e) the chest radiograph can show signs of left ventricular failure before it is recognisable clinically

E25   On a lateral cervical radiograph widening of preverebral soft tissues can occur in
(a) haemophilia
(b) trauma
(c) laryngomalacia
(d) tuberculosis
(e) sickle cell disease

E26   In Henoch–Schönlein purpura
(a) the patient is usually over 20 years of age
(b) gastrointestinal bleeding is a symptom
(c) mortality is greater than 50%
(d) in the majority red cells are present in the urine
(e) arthralgia is a symptom

E27   On a radioisotope bone scan
(a) there is increased uptake in hyperostosis frontalis interna
(b) increased activity can be present in successfully treated osteomyelitis
(c) increased uptake may occur in pulmonary and liver metastases from an osteoscarcoma
(d) a cartilage-capped exostosis will not show increased activity unless sarcomatous change has occurred
(e) increased activity can be seen in a primary neuroblastoma

E28   In dysthyroid exophthalmos
(a) plain radiographs of the orbit are normal
(b) typically CT will show thickening of the affected muscles
(c) orbital phlebography gives a characteristic appearance

(d) there may be associated periosteal new bone formation in the hands

(e) CT scan may show increased volume of intra-orbital fat

E29 The following associations can occur:

(a) duodenal obstruction and Christmas disease

(b) polycythaemia and cerebellar haemangioblastoma

(c) ACTH secretion and oat cell carcinoma of the bronchus

(d) alpha-1-antitrypsin deficiency and upper zone emphysematous change in the lung fields

(e) hypertension and diarrhoea

E30 In computerised tomography of the head

(a) calcification may be seen in lymphomatous deposits after irradiation

(b) circumferential enhancement with contrast by a low density lesion is diagnostic of a cerebral abscess

(c) dilatation of the lateral ventricles can be shown in sarcoidosis

(d) there is often calcification in acoustic neuromas

(e) there is enhancement of acute demyelinating plaques after injection of contrast medium.

E

Answers

E1
(a) **T**
(b) **F** upper zone changes in chronic stage, generalised or lower zone changes in acute stage
(c) **F** very rare
(d) **F**
(e) **F** leucocytosis with shift to left is normal

E2
(a) **T**
(b) **F** occurs in aortic valve
(c) **T**
(d) **T**
(e) **F** occurs in pericardium and mediastinal pleura

E3
(a) **T**
(b) **T**
(c) **T** Grieg's disease
(d) **F** sclerotic changes occur in the base of the skull
(e) **F**

E4
(a) **T**
(b) **F** hepatic fibrosis is associated with childhood-type of polycystic disease
(c) **F**
(d) **T** about 10% have intracranial aneurysms
(e) **T** about 10% develop stones

E5
(a) **F** xanthomatosis
(b) **T**
(c) **F** early infancy
(d) **T** punctate calcific foci in enlarged adrenal glands
(e) **T**

E6
(a) **T** due to calcification
(b) **F** rare—seen in thalassaemia

(c) **T** non-accidental injury, hypervitaminosis A
and cortical hyperostosis should also be excluded
(d) **T**
(e) **F** pigment stones

E7
(a) **T**
(b) **F**
(c) **T**
(d) **T** occurs in 5–10% of cases
(e) **T** due to necrosis

E8
(a) **T**
(b) **F**
(c) **F**
(d) **F**
(e) **T**

E9
(a) **T**
(b) **T**
(c) **T**
(d) **T**
(e) **F** raised

E10
(a) **T**
(b) **F**
(c) **T**
(d) **T** probably more frequent than total lung
involvement
(e) **F** without hypoxia there is no stimulus for
bronchial circulation to enlarge

E11
(a) **T** in the presence of atrial myxoma and
subacute bacterial endocarditis (SBE)
(b) **T** in the presence of atrial myxoma and SBE
(c) **T** in mitral stenosis
(d) **F**
(e) **T**

E12
(a) **T**
(b) **F**
(c) **F**
(d) **T** epiphyseal infarction can also occur
(e) **F** infarction occurs in epiphyses

E13
(a) **T**
(b) **T**

(c) **T** due to increased uptake by the spleen

(d) **F** there is a localised area of reduced activity

(e) **T** high activity is seen in the caudate lobe, which drains independently into the vena cava and retains its function

E14

(a) **F** three-quarters of cases before closure of epiphyses

(b) **T**

(c) **T**

(d) **F** can be extremely rapid in growth

(e) **F**

E15

(a) **T**

(b) **T**

(c) **T**

(d) **T** often the second and third

(e) **F** distal interphalangeal joints affected first

E16

(a) **T**

(b) **T**

(c) **F** congenital dilation of the bile ducts

(d) **T**

(e) **F**

E17

(a) **T**

(b) **T**

(c) **T** occasionally the left lung is plethoric too

(d) **F** not usually seen before the age of 10 years

(e) **T**

E18

(a) **T**

(b) **F**

(c) **T**

(d) **F**

(e) **T**

E19

(a) **T**

(b) **T** calcification is seen in about 6% of renal carcinomas

(c) **F** lactic dehydrogenase activity in urine increased

(d) **T**

(e) **T**

E20

(a) **T**

(b) **T**

(c) F

(d) F

(e) F in sigmoid only

E21

(a) T

(b) T

(c) T collapse of the lung may be delayed, if the bronchial tear is partial

(d) F distal aortic knuckle

(e) T

E22

(a) F benign ovarian fibroma can cause this

(b) F

(c) T

(d) F inflammatory mass can cause similar appearance

(e) T

E23

(a) T

(b) F occurs in trisomy 21

(c) T

(d) T

(e) T

E24

(a) T

(b) F redistribution of thallium can take three to four hours

(c) F

(d) T also on left ventriculography and echocardiography

(e) T

E25

(a) T

(b) T may not necessarily be associated with a fracture

(c) T

(d) T

(e) F

E26

(a) F usually less than 16 years old

(b) T

(c) F a self-limiting disease with good prognosis

(d) T

(e) T

E27

(a) T

(b) **T** due to continuing bone repair
(c) **T**
(d) **F** increased activity is not necessarily an indication of malignancy
(e) **T** seen in about one-third of cases

E28
(a) **F** increased soft tissue density and medial rectus enlargement can cause displacement of the medial orbital wall
(b) **T**
(c) **T** downward displacement of second part of the ophthalmic vein
(d) **T** thyroid acropachy. Seen after thyroidectomy
(e) **T**

E29
(a) **T** submucosal haemorrhage
(b) **T**
(c) **T**
(d) **F** lower zone emphysema
(e) **T** phaeochromocytoma and medullary carcinoma of the thyroid

E30
(a) **T**
(b) **F** identical appearance can be seen with a glioma
(c) **T**
(d) **F** very rare
(e) **T**

F

Questions

F1 Pneumomediastinum can be seen in
(a) legionnaires' disease
(b) ketoacidosis
(c) histiocytosis
(d) duodenal perforation
(e) respiratory distress syndrome

F2 Acoustic neuromas
(a) erode the crista transversalis
(b) are bilateral in 20% of cases
(c) occasionally contain calcium which can be visualised on computerised tomography
(d) rarely enhance with intravenous contrast
(e) occur in von Hippel–Lindau syndrome

F3 On a mammogram
(a) calcification is commonly widely distributed in sclerosing adenosis
(b) fibroadenomas can be seen without radiologically demonstrable calcification
(c) fine irregular calcification is seen in intraduct carcinoma
(d) large, flake-like, irregular calcification is an indication of benign disease
(e) eggshell calcification is seen in galactocoeles

F4 The following are features of scleroderma:
(a) antinuclear antibodies in the blood
(b) pneumoperitoneum
(c) narrowing of oesophago-gastric junction
(d) pericardial effusion
(e) loss of valvulae conniventes in the small bowel

F5 Cerebral calcification is a feature of
(a) congenital syphilis
(b) cytomegalic inclusion disease
(c) Alzheimer's syndrome
(d) Fanconi's syndrome
(e) toxoplasmosis

F6 Osteoid osteomas
(a) usually occur in middle-aged adults
(b) can be detected on radioisotope bone scanning

(c) are more common in males

(d) have a predilection for vertebral bodies

(e) rarely cause periosteal new bone formation in children

F7 Calcification in the pancreas may occur in

(a) cystadenoma

(b) hypoparathyroidism

(c) mumps

(d) malnutrition

(e) filariasis

F8 The following are correct:

(a) absent frontal sinuses are associated with persisting metopic suture

(b) sphenoid mucocoeles can cause internal carotid artery thrombosis

(c) Turner's syndrome is associated with absence of the frontal sinuses

(d) ethmoidal osteomas can cause spontaneous pneumocephalus

(e) anterior cranial meningocoeles can be indistinguishable from frontal mucocoeles on plain radiographs

F9 Calcification can occur in pulmonary metastases from

(a) carcinoma of the pancreas

(b) carcinoma of the breast

(c) adenocarcinoma of the thyroid

(d) squamous cell carcinoma

(e) papillary cystadenocarcinoma of the ovary

F10 Bone infarcts

(a) in dysbaric osteonecrosis are commonly juxta-articular

(b) occur in Gaucher's disease

(c) occur in thalassaemia major

(d) are often diaphyseal in sickle cell disease

(e) are seen in acute pancreatitis

F11 In the spine

(a) ependymomas are the commonest intramedullary tumour

(b) meningiomas usually occur in the lumbar region

(c) gliomas cause expansion

(d) calcification in neurofibomas can be seen on plain radiographs

(e) a chordoma producers a poorly defined area of bone destruction

F12 In osteomalacia

(a) a dorsal kyphosis is often present

(b) vertebral bodies may be biconcave
(c) there is a relative abundance of osteoid in the bone
(d) bone pain is unusual
(e) deformities disappear with adequate treatment

F13 Hepatosplenomegaly is seen in the following conditions:
(a) histiocytosis X
(b) myelosclerosis
(c) coeliac disease
(d) kala-azar
(e) thalassaemia

F14 Posterior vertebral body scalloping is seen in
(a) neurofibromatosis
(b) acromegaly
(c) aortic aneurysm
(d) Morquio's syndrome
(e) juvenile osteoporosis

F15 Lymphangiography
(a) is contraindicated in severe chronic bronchitis
(b) can fail to demonstrate heavily infiltrated nodes
(c) can demonstrate lymphocoeles in the pelvis
(d) can demonstrate involved inguinal nodes in teratoma of the testis
(e) can distinguish between tuberculous lymphadenitis and lymphoma

F16 With posterior dislocation of the shoulder
(a) the patient is able to rotate the humerus externally
(b) the glenohumeral joint can appear widened on the anteroposterior radiograph
(c) an associated impaction fracture involves the anterior part of the humeral head
(d) there is a likelihood of accompanying neuro-vascular injury
(e) recurrence is a common complication

F17 The heart can be shifted to the left on the PA radiograph with
(a) sternal depression
(b) complete pericardial defect
(c) ventriculoseptal defect
(d) complete situs inversus
(e) Marfan's syndrome

F18 The following are correct:
(a) in spinal stenosis the anteroposterior diameter of the lumbar spine canal is less than 15 mm.

(b) in spinal stenosis pain and weakness of the legs is precipitated by walking

(c) the plain radiographs in acute disc prolapse can be normal

(d) lateral prolapse of the lumbrosacral disc can cause compression of the first sacral nerve root

(e) in the cervical spine disc prolapse is most likely to occur at the C2–3 level

F19   In multiple myeloma
(a) the bone marrow contains abnormal lymphocytes
(b) there is lymph node enlargement
(c) alkaline phosphatase is usually elevated
(d) chronic renal failure occurs
(e) radioisotope bone scanning always shows the extent of the disease

F20   Gas in the portal venous system
(a) appears on ultrasound examination as brightly echogenic foci within the liver
(b) is seen on plain radiographs as branching lucencies extending to the periphery of the liver
(c) is associated with necrotising enterocolitis in infants
(d) is a known complication of double contrast barium enema in patients with active ulcerative colitis
(e) is associated with 100% mortality rate

F21   Sacroiliitis is seen in the following:
(a) Whipple's disease
(b) sarcoidosis
(c) Reiter's syndrome
(d) Behçet's disease
(e) psoriasis

F22   In echocardiography systolic anterior motion of the anterior mitral valve leaflet occurs in
(a) hypertrophic obstructive cardiomyopathy
(b) aortic incompetence
(c) beri beri heart failure
(d) ASD
(e) VSD

F23   Pseudomyxomatous peritonitis occurs with
(a) ovarian fibroma
(b) cholangiocarcinoma
(c) neuroenteric cysts
(d) Meckel's diverticulum
(e) mucocoele of the appendix

F24   Pulmonary artery stenosis
(a) is associated with the fetal alcohol syndrome

(b) is associated with infantile hypercalcaemia
(c) is inherited as an autosomal recessive with variable penetrance
(d) occurs in the carcinoid syndrome
(e) is associated with bicuspid aortic valves

F25 Terminal phalangeal sclerosis is associated with
(a) rheumatoid arthritis
(b) tuberculosis
(c) sarcoidosis
(d) pleural fibroma
(e) chronic active hepatitis

F26 The following are associated with focal absent activity on splenic scintigraphy
(a) septic emboli
(b) cyanotic heart disease
(c) trauma
(d) sarcoidosis
(e) thalassaemia

F27 Hypercalcaemia is seen in
(a) renal tubular acidosis
(b) sarcoidosis
(c) multiple myeloma
(d) Addison's disease
(e) scleroderma

F28 In a child a filling defect in the bladder at intravenous urography can be due to
(a) rhabdomyosarcoma
(b) a phaeochromocytoma
(c) an ectopic ureterocoele
(d) posterior urethral valves
(e) schistosomal infection

F29 Sclerosis of orbital walls occurs in
(a) histiocytosis X
(b) polyostotic fibrous dysplasia
(c) hyperostosis frontalis interna
(d) intraorbital glioma
(e) intraorbital dermoid

F30 Ankylosing spondylitis
(a) occasionally only involves one sacroiliac joint
(b) is associated with femoral hernia
(c) is associated with mitral regurgitation
(d) is associated with iritis
(e) is associated with apical pulmonary fibrosis

Answers

F1
(a) **F**
(b) **T**
(c) **T**
(d) **T**
(e) **T**

F2
(a) **T**
(b) **F** only a few cases are bilateral
(c) **T**
(d) **F**
(e) **F**

F3
(a) **T**
(b) **T**
(c) **T**
(d) **F** Seen occasionally in mucoid carcinoma and cystosarcoma phylloides. Benign calcification is smooth
(e) **T**

F4
(a) **T**
(b) **T** due to pneumatosis intestinalis
(c) **F** oesophago-gastric junction becomes patulous
(d) **F**
(e) **F**

F5
(a) **F**
(b) **T** fine nodular calcification in the dilated ventricular walls
(c) **F**
(d) **F**
(e) **T** flecks of calcification in cortex and streaks in the basal ganglia

F6
(a) **F** teenagers and young adults
(b) **T**

(c) **T**
(d) **F** neural arch is the usual site of vertebral involvement
(e) **F** especially florid reaction in children

F7
(a) **T**
(b) **F**
(c) **F**
(d) **T**
(e) **F**

F8
(a) **T**
(b) **T**
(c) **F**
(d) **T**
(e) **T**

F9
(a) **T**
(b) **T**
(c) **T**
(d) **F**
(e) **T**

F10
(a) **T** especially proximal humerus and femur
(b) **T**
(c) **F**
(d) **T** can mimic acute pyogenic osteomyelitis
(e) **T**

F11
(a) **T**
(b) **F** thoracic
(c) **F**
(d) **F** neurofibromas do not calcify
(e) **F** slow growing and defect well-defined

F12
(a) **T**
(b) **T**
(c) **T** characteristic abnormality in the bone
(d) **F** aches and pains are amongst the earliest signs
(e) **F**

F13
(a) **T**
(b) **T**
(c) **F** small spleen
(d) **T**
(e) **T**

F14
- (a) **T**
- (b) **T**
- (c) **F** the anterior surface
- (d) **F**
- (e) **F**

F15
- (a) **T**
- (b) **T**
- (c) **T** there is pooling of oily contrast medium
- (d) **T** secondary to scrotal involvement
- (e) **F** appearance can be identical

F16
- (a) **F** the humeral head is in fixed internal rotation
- (b) **T** due to lateral displacement of the humeral head, but there is more usually overlap of the glenoid and humerus
- (c) **T** shown on the axillary view
- (d) **F** this occurs in anterior dislocation which stretches the neurovascular bundle
- (e) **F** recurrence is rare. Usually in patients who have spontaneous dislocation

F17
- (a) **T**
- (b) **T**
- (c) **F**
- (d) **F**
- (e) **F**

F18
- (a) **T**
- (b) **T** known as intermittent claudication of cauda equina
- (c) **T**
- (d) **F** L5 nerve root
- (e) **F** discs between C5, 6 and 7 are most likely to prolapse

F19
- (a) **F** there is proliferation of plasma cells
- (b) **F**
- (c) **F** this can rise if pathological fracture occurs
- (d) **T**
- (e) **F** the majority of bone lesions in multiple myeloma excite little or no new bone formation and radiographs are more helpful

F20
- (a) **T**

(b) **T**

(c) **T**

(d) **T**

(e) **F** not a fatal sign in infants and following barium enema the prognosis is good. Poor prognosis if secondary to infarction of bowel, infection or ulceration

F21

(a) **T**

(b) **F**

(c) **T** tends to be asymmetrical

(d) **T** tends to be asymmetrical

(e) **T** occurs in 40% of cases

F22

(a) **T**

(b) **T**

(c) **T** high output failure

(d) **F**

(e) **F**

F23

(a) **T**

(b) **F**

(c) **F**

(d) **F**

(e) **T**

F24

(a) **F** rubella syndrome

(b) **T**

(c) **F** autosomal dominant

(d) **T** due to thickening of the pulmonary valve

(e) **F**

F25

(a) **T** may precede onset of joint symptoms by many years

(b) **F**

(c) **T**

(d) **F** causes hypertrophic pulmonary osteo-arthropathy

(e) **T**

F26

(a) **T**

(b) **T**

(c) **T**

(d) **T**

(e) **F**

F27
- (a) **T**
- (b) **T**
- (c) **T**
- (d) **F**
- (e) **F**

F28
- (a) **T**
- (b) **T**
- (c) **T**
- (d) **F**
- (e) **T**

F29
- (a) **T**   but uncommon
- (b) **T**
- (c) **F**   involves skull vault only
- (d) **F**
- (e) **F**   causes bone destruction

F30
- (a) **T**
- (b) **F**   inguinal hernia
- (c) **F**   aortic incompetence
- (d) **T**   about 25%
- (e) **T**

G

Questions

G1 The following are features of allergic broncho-pulmonary aspergillosis:
(a) episodic asthma
(b) elevated serum IgE levels
(c) proximal bronchiectasis
(d) peripheral eosinophilia
(e) a cavitating mass on chest radiograph

G2 Enterogenous cysts of the central nervous system
(a) are associated with tracheo-oesophageal fistulae
(b) can occur at any level in the spine
(c) are always extramedullary
(d) are associated with anterior spinal defects
(e) can cause localised widening of the interpedicular distance

G3 Mediastinal lymph node enlargement is seen in
(a) pneumoconiosis
(b) erythema nodosum
(c) infectious mononucleosis
(d) miliary tuberculosis
(e) legionnaires' disease

G4 A choledochal cyst
(a) can present as a painless mass
(b) commonly presents in the neonate
(c) is more common in males than in females
(d) is demonstrated on a technetium-99m colloid liver scan
(e) is associated with an increased incidence of cholangiocarcinoma

G5 In subarachnoid haemorrhage
(a) haematoma in the corpus callosum on the CT scan is an indication of bleeding from the anterior cerebral artery
(b) extravasated blood will be demonstrated in the majority of cases by CT scanning in the first week after haemorrhage
(c) there is an association with polycystic kidneys

- (d) communicating hydrocephalus rarely develops before 72 hours
- (e) the commonest cause is a ruptured aneurysm

G6 Periosteal reactions can be seen in
- (a) multiple myeloma
- (b) actinomycosis
- (c) infantile cortical hyperostosis
- (d) osteoid osteoma
- (e) syphilis

G7 The following are causes of anterior mediastinal masses:
- (a) thymic tumour
- (b) teratodermoid tumour
- (c) bronchogenic cysts
- (d) pericardial cyst
- (e) hernia through the foramen of Bochdalek

G8 The following are extrapulmonary manifestations of carcinoma of the bronchus:
- (a) peripheral neuropathy
- (b) thrombocytopenic purpura
- (c) dermatomyositis
- (d) Behçet's syndrome
- (e) Sjögren's syndrome

G9 The kidneys are characteristically enlarged in
- (a) chronic pyelonephritis
- (b) uraemic medullary cystic disease
- (c) polycystic disease
- (d) acute renal venous thrombosis
- (e) lymphoma

G10 On a perfusion lung scan diminished activity can occur in the left lower lobe with
- (a) bronchial carcinoma
- (b) mitral stenosis
- (c) bronchial adenoma
- (d) bronchogenic cyst
- (e) scimitar syndrome

G11 Coarctation of the aorta
- (a) is commonly preductal if presentation occurs in the first year of life
- (b) is often associated with bicuspid aortic valve
- (c) can be associated with soft tissue shadowing behind the sternum on lateral chest radiographs
- (d) is associated with atrial septal defect
- (e) is more common in females

G12 Atrophy of the distal phalanges occurs in
- (a) epidermolysis bullosa

- (b) ergot poisoning
- (c) carbon tetrachloride poisoning
- (d) systemic lupus erythematosis
- (e) pseudoxanthoma elasticum

G13 When the abdomen is examined by computerised tomography
- (a) air introduced at operation on the aorta may still be present in the retroperitoneal tissues in the second week
- (b) enlargement of the inferior vena cava is characteristically seen in caval thrombosis
- (c) normal pancreatic tissue shows marked enhancement after intravenous contract
- (d) cysts in the tail of the pancreas may be seen distal to a carcinoma
- (e) the renal veins cannot be identified after injection of contrast

G14 On ultrasound examination of the female pelvis
- (a) fibromyomas can be seen in 60% of patients over the age of 35 years
- (b) malignant change in fibromyomas is suspected if the uterine midline echo is absent
- (c) in most cases of hydatidiform mole there is a highly echogenic pelvic mass
- (d) an incomplete abortion can mimic trophoblastic disease
- (e) bilateral multiloculated ovarian cysts are commonly associated with hydatidiform moles

G15 Calcification of the pinna is seen in
- (a) onchronosis
- (b) frost bite
- (c) gout
- (d) Addion's disease
- (e) scleroderma

G16 When the spine is injured
- (a) in the majority of cases manifestations of cord injury occur late
- (b) spinal cord injury occurs without radiographic evidence of fractures in 50% of cases
- (c) atlanto-occipital dislocation is rarely accompanied by neurological abnormalities
- (d) fracture of the posterior arch of C2 is rarely associated with neurological abnormalities
- (e) the central spinal cord injury syndrome is associated with hyperextension injuries of the cervical spine

G17 In the gallbladder

(a) large smooth radiolucent stones are unlikely to respond to dissolution with oral chenodeoxycholic acid

(b) calcification in the walls is associated with an increased incidence of carcinoma

(c) gas-containing gallstones are associated with emphysematous cholecystitis

(d) adenomyomatosis does not cause symptoms unless stones are present

(e) cholesterosis is a cause of filling defects around the neck on oral cholecystography

G18 The following are correct:

(a) avascular necrosis is known to occur after fracture of the talus

(b) premature fusion of a slipped epiphysis can occur

(c) in a Salter type 1 epiphyseal injury there is separation of the epiphysis with adjacent metaphyseal fragment

(d) Salter type V epiphyseal injuries have an increased rate of premature fusion

(e) fractures of the mandible commonly occur in the region of the canine teeth

G19 Phaeochromocytomas

(a) are associated with medullary carcinoma of the thyroid

(b) are associated with neurofibromatosis

(c) produce excessive serotonin

(d) can be demonstrated by scanning 30 minutes after injection of radiolabelled MIBG (meta-iodo-benzo-guanidine)

(e) are extra-suprarenal in 10% of cases

G20 Plethoric lung fields in a cyanosed infant are seen in

(a) truncus anteriosus

(b) tricuspid atresia without pulmonary stenosis

(c) scimitar syndrome

(d) complete transposition of the great vessels

(e) Fallot's tetralogy

G21 Pigmented villonodular synovitis

(a) most frequently occurs in patients over the age of 50

(b) can involve any synovial joint

(c) frequently calcifies

(d) produces dense nodular soft tissue swelling on the radiograph

(e) commonly progresses to malignant synovioma

G22 Schistosomal infection produces
- (a) polypoidal lesion in the distal colon
- (b) paraplegia
- (c) pulmonary arterial hypertension
- (d) oesophageal varices
- (e) hilar lymphadenopathy

G23 In acute lympathic leukaemia
- (a) sternal involvement is common
- (b) splenic enlargement often occurs
- (c) dense metaphyseal lines occur
- (d) metaphyseal erosions of the humerus are seen
- (e) osteosclerosis can occur after therapy

G24 Necrotising enterocolitis
- (a) is first detected by gas in the bowel wall on plain radiographs
- (b) occurs after umbilical catheterisation
- (c) is associated with respiratory distress syndrome
- (d) is associated with cystic fibrosis
- (e) causes strictures in the long term

G25 When the scaphoid is fractured
- (a) the proximal pole is most commonly involved
- (b) non-union is most common with fractures of the proximal pole
- (c) a radioisotope bone scan may be positive with a normal radiograph
- (d) healing occurs without radiologically visible periosteal callus
- (e) a fracture of the radial styloid process should be sought

G26 In cystic fibrosis
- (a) the majority of patients present with meconium ileus
- (b) scrotal calcification can be seen on a radiograph of a neonate
- (c) a micro-gallbladder is often present
- (d) pancreatic calcification is present in 50% of patients
- (e) rectal prolapse occurs

C27 Lymphangitis carcinomatosa is typically a feature of
- (a) carcinoma of the thyroid
- (b) carcinoma of the bronchus
- (c) hepatoma
- (d) hypernephroma
- (e) carcinoma of the pancreas

G28 **Widening of the superior orbital fissure may be seen with**
(a) aqueduct stenosis
(b) aneurysm of the internal carotid artery
(c) eosinophilic granuloma
(d) neurofibromatosis
(e) pituitary adenoma

G29 **In a patient who has acid-fast bacilli in the urine**
(a) calcification of the bladder is common
(b) bladder disease is associated with extensive renal disease
(c) ureteric involvement causes shortening of the ureters
(d) renal disease can produce changes identical to reflux nephropathy
(e) ureteric calculi are commonly present

G30 **In the spine**
(a) spina bifida is most commonly seen at L2/3
(b) sacral agenesis occurs in babies of diabetic mothers
(c) diastematomyelia is associated with widening of the interpedicular distance
(d) bony abnormality on plain films is not frequently seen with anterior sacral meningocoeles
(e) narrowing of the disc space can be the earliest sign of tuberculous infection

G

Answers

G1
(a) **T**
(b) **T**
(c) **T**
(d) **T**
(e) **F** pulmonary aspergilloma

G2
(a) **F**
(b) **T** especially lower cervical and upper thoracic region
(c) **F** are occasionally intramedullary
(d) **F** this is seen with extraspinal enterogenous cysts
(e) **T** there are not always plain film signs

G3
(a) **F**
(b) **T**
(c) **T**
(d) **F**
(e) **F**

G4
(a) **T**
(b) **F** child under 10 years of age
(c) **F** females to males 4:1
(d) **F** choledochal cysts are demonstrated on HIDA scans
(e) **T**

G5
(a) **T**
(b) **T**
(c) **T**
(d) **F** can develop rapidly due to blood and clot obstructing the CSF flow
(e) **T**

G6
(a) **F**
(b) **T** characteristic. Especially mandible and ribs

(c) **T** extensive periosteal new bone along margins of long bones

(d) **T**

(e) **T**

G7

(a) **T**

(b) **T**

(c) **F** middle mediastinum

(d) **T** usually right sided

(e) **F** posterior

G8

(a) **T**

(b) **T**

(c) **T**

(d) **F**

(e) **F**

G9

(a) **F** the kidney becomes small and irregularly scarred

(b) **F** may be large or small depending on number of cysts and degree of fibrosis

(c) **T**

(d) **T**

(e) **F**

G10

(a) **T**

(b) **T** collapse of left lower lobe

(c) **T** causing ostruction of left lower lobe bronchus

(d) **T**

(e) **F**

G11

(a) **T**

(b) **T** occurs frequently with post-ductal coarctation

(c) **T** due to dilatation of internal mammary artery

(d) **F**

(e) **F** if seen in females Turner's syndrome should be suspected

G12

(a) **T**

(b) **T**

(c) **F**

(d) **F**

(e) **T**

G13

(a) **T**

(b) **T** but not always
(c) **T** to 50–80 Hounsfield units
(d) **T** retention cysts due to duct obstruction
(e) **F**

G14
(a) **F** 10–20%
(b) **F** not possible to differentiate from normal fibroids
(c) **F** less than 5%
(d) **T**
(e) **T**

G15
(a) **T**
(b) **T** commonest cause
(c) **T**
(d) **T**
(e) **F**

G16
(a) **F** about 85% of cases present immediately
(b) **F** 10% do not have a fracture
(c) **F** almost invariably fatal
(d) **T**
(e) **T** central spinal cord injury syndrome is composed of motor signs greater in the upper than the lower limbs, bladder dysfunction and varying sensory loss below the level of the lesion

G17
(a) **F** these are usually rich in cholesterol and likely to respond
(b) **T**
(c) **F**
(d) **F**
(e) **T**

G18
(a) **T**
(b) **T**
(c) **F** type 1 is complete separation of the epiphysis
(d) **T** compression injury to the growth plate
(e) **T**

G19
(a) **T**
(b) **T**
(c) **F** catecholamines
(d) **F** 24 hours after injection
(e) **T**

G20
- (a) **T**
- (b) **T**
- (c) **F** seen with total anomalous venous drainage
- (d) **T**
- (e) **F** oligaemic lung fields and infants are rarely cyanosed

G21
- (a) **F** occurs in adolescents and young to middle-aged adults
- (b) **T**
- (c) **F** very rare. If there is calcification a malignant synovioma should be considered
- (d) **T** due to haemosiderin content the swelling is unusually dense
- (e) **F** malignant change extremely rare

G22
- (a) **T**
- (b) **T**
- (c) **T**
- (d) **T**
- (e) **F**

G23
- (a) **F**
- (b) **F**
- (c) **T**
- (d) **T** medial surface of humeral shaft
- (e) **T** also as a primary manifestation

G24
- (a) **F** first sign is atonic segments of bowel
- (b) **T**
- (c) **T**
- (d) **F**
- (e) **T**

G25
- (a) **F** the waist 70%, the distal pole 10%
- (b) **T**
- (c) **T**
- (d) **T** healed by endosteal callus
- (e) **T** fractures of the capitate and triquetrum also occur, as does peri-lunate dislocation

G26
- (a) **F** respiratory problems
- (b) **T**
- (c) **T**
- (d) **F** less than 10%
- (d) **T**

G27

- (a) **F**
- (b) **T**
- (c) **F**
- (d) **F**
- (e) **T**

G28

- (a) **F** thinning of the wings of the sphenoid
- (b) **T**
- (c) **F** clear-cut erosions in the greater wing of the sphenoid
- (d) **T**
- (e) **T**

G29

- (a) **F** calcification is seen in kidneys, seminal vesicle and prostate but only occasionally in the bladder
- (b) **T**
- (c) **T** ureters shorten and enter bladder perpendicularly, causing 'golf hole' appearance
- (d) **T**
- (e) **F** uncommon. Seen in schistosomiasis

G30

- (a) **F** L5/S1
- (b) **T**
- (c) **T**
- (d) **F** there is a well-defined defect of the sacrum
- (e) **T**

H

Questions

H1 In fibrous dysplasia
(a) continued enlargement of affected bone in adult life is a recognised feature
(b) malignant change is rare
(c) polyostotic lesions are associated with precocious puberty
(d) there is an association with hyperparathyroidism
(e) the alkaline phosphatase is elevated

H2 Protein-losing enteropathy occurs with
(a) gastrointestinal lymphoma
(b) Menetrier's disease
(c) Whipple's disease
(d) constrictive pericarditis
(e) hypothyroidism

H3 Nephrotic syndrome may occur in
(a) renal vein thrombosis
(b) Henoch–Schönlein pupura
(c) gold therapy
(d) secondary amyloidosis
(e) neurofibromatosis

H4 In the foot
(a) tarso-metatarsal dislocation occurs in diabetics without a history of significant trauma
(b) avascular necrosis usually affects the head of the second metatarsal
(c) the distal component of a sub-talar dislocation is most commonly displaced laterally
(d) avascular necrosis of the distal fragment of the talus may occur after a fracture
(e) after compression fracture of the calcaneum Boehler's angle may be normal

H5 Sclerosing cholangitis
(a) is associated with Crohn's disease
(b) is commonly associated with anti-mitochondrial antibodies in the blood
(c) does not involve the extra-hepatic ducts
(d) produces multiple strictures and beading of the intrahepatic ducts

(e) has non-filling of the gallbladder as a diagnostic feature at retrograde endoscopic cholangiography

H6 In allergic maxillary sinusitis
(a) mucosal thickening tends to be scalloped
(b) fluid levels are more common than in infective sinusitis
(c) involvement of the other sinuses is unusual
(d) polyp formation is unusual
(e) thickening of the nasal turbinates occurs

H7 Ewing's tumour
(a) is most commonly seen in patients less than 30 years old
(b) does not occur in flat bones
(c) causes characteristic layering of the periosteum
(d) often metastasises elsewhere in the skeleton
(e) has a histological appearance very similar to neuroblastoma

H8 Emphysematous changes in the lung fields are associated with
(a) Marfan's syndrome
(b) alpha-1-antitrypsin deficiency
(c) pulmonary artery stenosis
(d) sinusitis
(e) McLeod's syndrome

H9 In endometriosis
(a) calcification can be seen on plain abdominal radiographs
(b) rectal bleeding commonly occurs as a presenting symptom
(c) there is an increased incidence of endometrial carcinoma
(d) retroperitoneal fibrosis can occur
(e) the patient can be postmenopausal at presentation

H10 In Klebsiella pneumonia
(a) the lower lobe is affected more frequently than the upper lobe
(b) haemoptysis is common
(c) resolution is usually complete after treatment
(d) blood culture is usually positive
(e) bulging of the adjacent fissure is characteristic

H11 In Noonan's syndrome
(a) horseshoe kidneys occur
(b) the chromosomes are normal
(c) the fourth metacarpal is short
(d) the commonest cardiac anomaly is pulmonary stenosis
(e) webbing of the neck occurs

H12 **On ultrasound examination of the pregnant uterus**
(a) the placenta can be identified at 12 weeks' gestation
(b) a crown–rump measurement is commonly used between 8 and 12 weeks' gestation to assess fetal maturity
(c) biparietal measurements are most accurate after 32 weeks' gestation
(d) a fetal sac can be visualised at 3 weeks' gestation
(e) the fetal heart pulsation is rarely seen before 12 weeks

H13 **On a chest radiograph an enlarged azygos vein is associated with**
(a) alcoholic cirrhosis
(b) left ventricular failure
(c) renal cell carcinoma
(d) asplenia
(e) retroperitoneal fibrosis

H14 **Diabetes mellitus is associated with**
(a) acromegaly
(b) cystadenoma of the pancreas
(c) hypothyroidism
(d) hypopituitarism
(e) hyperparathyroidism

H15 **In pulmonary arterio-venous aneurysms**
(a) the size of the lesion indicates the size of the shunt
(b) phleboliths can be present
(c) there is an association with mucocutaneous haemangiomata
(d) paradoxical embolus can be the presenting feature
(e) the diagnosis is usually initially confirmed by tomography

H16 **Predominantly interstitial pulmonary oedema is seen in**
(a) acute myocardial infarction
(b) persistent left ventricular failure
(c) severe mitral stenosis
(d) opiate overdose
(e) adult respiratory distress syndrome

H17 **In hepatoma**
(a) the ultrasound appearance is diagnostic
(b) there is increased uptake on technetium-99m colloid liver scan

(c) there is increased uptake of gallium-67 by the tumour

(d) the alpha-fetoprotein level is high

(e) hepatitis A is a known predisposing factor

H18 Calcification in the basal ganglia can occur in

(a) Fahr's syndrome

(b) Sturge–Weber syndrome

(c) toxoplasmosis

(d) hypoparathyroidism

(e) hyperparathyroidism

H19 Causes of bile-stained vomiting in a neonate are

(a) meconium plug

(b) septicaemia

(c) choledochal cyst

(d) Hirshsprung's disease

(e) malrotation of the bowel

H20 In calcium pyrophosphate deposition disease

(a) there is calcification of the fibrocartilage of the public symphysis

(b) the articular cartilage of the interphalangeal joints is commonly calcified

(c) calcification is commonly present in the triangular cartilage of the distal radio-ulnar joint

(d) the serum calcium is elevated during an acute attack

(e) crystals of calcium pyrophosphate can be found in asymptomatic joints

H21 Enlargement of a jugular foramen is caused by

(a) neurofibromatosis

(b) metastatic deposits

(c) craniopharyngioma

(d) glomus jugulare tumour

(e) aneurysm of the basilar artery

H22 In neonatal cerebral ultrasound examination

(a) intraventricular haemorrhage is seen primarily in the matrix overlying the caudate nucleus

(b) fresh haemorrhage is indicated by bright echogenic areas

(c) presence of the septum cavum often indicates raised intracranial pressure (ICP)

(d) hydrocephalus is a complication of intraventricular haemorrhage

(e) a leptomeningeal cyst is seen as a late complication of intraventricular haemorrhage

H23 Abdominal aortic aneurysms

(a) involve the right iliac artery in 75% of cases

(b) involve the renal arteries in 90% of cases
(c) should not be demonstrated by femoral arteriography
(d) are associated with polyarteritis nodosa
(e) can predispose to retroperitoneal fibrosis

H24 Wegener's granulomatosis
(a) is commoner in females than males
(b) is associated with deafness
(c) usually produces hilar lymphadenopathy
(d) can have a relatively good prognosis if confined to the lungs
(e) can cause hypertension

H25 Renal cortical calcification occurs in
(a) Sheehan's syndrome
(b) acute tubular necrosis
(c) hyperoxaluria
(d) homocystinuria
(e) haemophilia

H26 In a patient with an amoebic abscess in the liver
(a) the abscess is commonly in the left lobe
(b) there is commonly a history of diarrhoea
(c) the appearance on ultrasound examination is characteristic
(d) calcification of the abscess wall is unusual
(e) amoebae are commonly found in the stools

H27 Rickets due to dietary deficiency
(a) does not affect the age of appearance of the epiphyses in the child
(b) produces bone abnormalities similar to those seen in Fanconi's syndrome
(c) commonly produces metaphyseal fractures
(d) causes narrowing of the zone of provisional calcification
(e) produces subperiosteal haematomas

H28 In Hirschsprung's disease
(a) there may be involvement of small bowel
(b) patients sometimes present with diarrhoea
(c) there is an association with duodenal atresia
(d) Gastrografin enemas are contraindicated
(e) the incidence is higher in children of diabetic mothers

H29 Osteochondritis dissecans can occur in the
(a) trochlea
(b) talus
(c) scaphoid

- (d) ulnar styloid
- (e) spinous process of C7

H30 **Columnar cell mucosa in the lower oesophagus**
- (a) is associated with chronic gastro-oesophageal reflux
- (b) can be shown on double contrast barium study
- (c) is associated with increased risk of squamous carcinoma
- (d) is associated with increased incidence of peptic ulceration of the oesophagus
- (e) can be demonstrated by isotope scanning with sodium pertechnetate

H

Answers

H1
(a) **T**
(b) **T**
(c) **T** Albright's syndrome
(d) **F**
(e) **F**

H2
(a) **T**
(b) **T**
(c) **T**
(d) **T**
(e) **F**

H3
(a) **T**
(b) **T**
(c) **T**
(d) **T**
(e) **F**

H4
(a) **T**
(b) **T** Freiberg's osteochondritis
(c) **F** medial displacement
(d) **F** proximal fragment
(e) **T**

H5
(a) **T** also associated with ulcerative colitis
(b) **F** usually absent
(c) **F** affects both intra- and extra-hepatic ducts
(d) **T**
(e) **F**

H6
(a) **T**
(b) **F**
(c) **F**
(d) **F**
(e) **T**

H7
(a) **T**

(b) **F** about half occur in flat bones, especially the innominate bone
(c) **T**
(d) **T**
(e) **T** can also look like reticulum cell sarcoma and anaplastic carcinoma

H8
(a) **T**
(b) **T**
(c) **F**
(d) **F**
(e) **T**

H9
(a) **F**
(b) **F**
(c) **F** sarcomatous changes
(d) **F** hydronephrosis results from ureteric deposits
(e) **T**

H10
(a) **F** no difference
(b) **T**
(c) **F**
(d) **F**
(e) **T**

H11
(a) **F** occur in Turner's syndrome
(b) **T** Turner phenotype and normal karyotope in all patients
(c) **F** occurs in Turner's syndrome. There may be clindactyly of fifth finger
(d) **T**
(e) **T** in this and Turner's syndrome

H12
(a) **T**
(b) **T**
(c) **F** become very inaccurate after 32 weeks
(d) **F** not usually seen before 5 or 6 weeks
(e) **F** Can be identified soon after the gestational sac is seen

H13
(a) **T**
(b) **T**
(c) **T** inferior vena caval obstruction
(d) **F** seen in polysplenia which is associated with IVC absence
(e) **T**

H14
(a)	**T**	in about 10%
(b)	**F**	
(c)	**T**	autoimmune thyroiditis
(d)	**F**	
(e)	**F**	

H15
(a)	**F**	
(b)	**T**	
(c)	**T**	Osler–Weber–Rendu syndrome
(d)	**T**	
(e)	**T**	the supplying vessels are demonstrated

H16
(a)	**F**	intra-alveolar oedema occurs
(b)	**T**	due to chronic elevation of pulmonary venous pressure
(c)	**T**	
(d)	**F**	
(e)	**F**	

H17
(a)	**F**	echo pattern indistinguishable from metastases
(b)	**F**	
(c)	**T**	
(d)	**T**	
(e)	**F**	hepatitis B

H18
(a)	**T**	
(b)	**F**	calcification lies on the surface of the brain
(c)	**T**	
(d)	**T**	
(e)	**T**	

H19
(a)	**T**	
(b)	**T**	
(c)	**F**	
(d)	**T**	
(e)	**T**	

H20
(a)	**F**	
(b)	**F**	calcification usually in articular cartilage of major joints
(c)	**T**	
(d)	**F**	elevated in hyperparathyroidism
(e)	**T**	

H21
(a)	**T**	

(b) **T**
(c) **F**
(d) **T**
(e) **F**

H22

(a) **T**
(b) **T**
(c) **F** its absence indicates raised ICP
(d) **T**
(e) **F**

H23

(a) **F**
(b) **F** only about 5%
(c) **F**
(d) **F**
(e) **T**

H24

(a) **F** about 2:1 males to females
(b) **T** due to eustachian tube involvement or otitis media
(c) **F**
(d) **T**
(e) **F** unlike polyarteritis

H25

(a) **T**
(b) **T**
(c) **T**
(d) **F**
(e) **F** although papillary necrosis can occur

H26

(a) **F** usually the right lobe
(b) **F**
(c) **F** pyogenic and amoebic abscesses have similar appearances
(d) **T**
(e) **F**

H27

(a) **F** they are delayed and smaller than usual
(b) **T** renal tubular deficiency. Phosphate, glucose and aminoacids are excreted in the urine
(c) **F**
(d) **T**
(e) **F** occur in vitamin C deficiency

H28

(a) **T**
(b) **T** spurious diarrhoea

(c)   **T**   Down's syndrome
(d)   **F**
(e)   **F**   microcolon in these children

129
(a)   **T**
(b)   **T**
(c)   **F**
(d)   **F**
(e)   **F**

130
(a)   **T**
(b)   **T**
(c)   **F**   adenocarcinoma
(d)   **T**
(e)   **T**

I

Questions

I1 Primary hyperparathyroidism
(a) is most commonly caused by parathyroid glandular hyperplasia
(b) is accompanied by polyuria
(c) rarely causes renal stones
(d) is associated with adenoma of the pancreas
(e) is confirmed by the loss of lamina dura around the teeth

I2 Diabetes insipidus and widespread interstitial changes in the lung fields are seen in
(a) systemic lupus erythematosus
(b) histiocytosis X
(c) biliary cirrhosis
(d) sarcoidosis
(e) tuberous sclerosis

I3 In hypertrophic cardiomyopathy
(a) there is often a significant family history
(b) cardiac enlargement is usually seen on the chest radiograph at presentation
(c) left ventricular outflow tract obstruction is always present
(d) enlargement of the coronary arteries is commonly seen on angiography
(e) there is often mitral regurgitation

I4 On ultrasound examination of the pregnant uterus
(a) placenta praevia is more easily seen with posteriorly sited placentas
(b) the placental position does not change after 28 weeks' gestation
(c) duodenal atresia in the fetus has a characteristic appearance.
(d) a 'halo' appearance of the fetal scalp is associated with maternal diabetes
(e) the fetal kidneys can be identified after 15 weeks' gestation

I5 In legionnaires' disease
(a) the hilar nodes are enlarged

- (b) associated abdominal symptoms are a feature
- (c) bilateral pleural effusions are characteristic
- (d) the diagnosis is usually confirmed by the detection of *Legionella pneumophila* in the sputum
- (e) treatment is with co-trimoxazole

I6 An osteosarcoma
- (a) usually occurs between 10 and 25 years
- (b) rarely extends into a joint
- (c) can cause ossifying metastases in the lungs
- (d) can be a complication of diaphyseal aclasia
- (e) is typically seen as a purely destructive lesion on the radiograph

I7 The following are recognised features of xanthogranulomatous pyelonephritis:
- (a) non-functioning kidney on intravenous urography
- (b) the presence of renal calculi
- (c) bilateral renal involvement
- (d) positive urine culture
- (e) a diagnostic circulatory pattern on renal angiography

I8 Pleural calcification occurs with exposure to
- (a) beryllium
- (b) haematite
- (c) talc
- (d) asbestos
- (e) barium

I9 The following are correct:
- (a) a significant amount of gallium-67 is excreted in breast milk
- (b) uptake of gallium-67 in hilar lymph nodes is diagnostic of lymphoma
- (c) focal increased uptake of gallium-67 in the liver can be due to metastatic melanoma
- (d) after injection of gallium-67 the first scan is done about six hours later
- (e) cerebral infarcts can accumulate gallium-67

I10 Fragmentation of the epiphyses can be seen in
- (a) hypothyroidism
- (b) chondroectodermal dysplasia
- (c) osteopetrosis
- (d) sickle cell anaemia
- (e) scurvy

I11 Bilateral pleural effusions
- (a) are usually present in acute extrinsic allergic alveolitis

(b) are a feature of adult respiratory distress syndrome
(c) are commonly seen in lymphoma
(d) are associated with benign ovarian fibroma
(e) are a characteristic feature of scleroderma

I12 In the nail-patella syndrome
(a) renal function is normal
(b) iliac horns are present
(c) inheritance is autosomal dominant
(d) the patellae are always absent
(e) the elbows are normal

I13 Mediastinal lymphadenopathy and bony abnormality of the hands are seen in the following
(a) Maffucci's syndrome
(b) sarcoidosis
(c) berylliosis
(d) scleroderma
(e) bronchogenic carcinoma

I14 On radiological examination of the parotid gland
(a) about 20% of calculi are opaque
(b) the ducts are dilated in Sjögren's syndrome
(c) the intraglandular ducts dilate when there is stenosis of the orifice of the duct
(d) sialectasis occurs in viral parotitis
(e) a mixed salivary tumour causes displacement of the intraglandular ducts

I15 HLA B27 antigen is associated with
(a) Reiter's syndrome
(b) Behçet's disease
(c) haemochromatosis
(d) Wilson's disease
(e) psoriasis

I16 In a child, pneumatocoele formation is seen in
(a) *Escherichia coli* pneumonia
(b) streptococcal pneumonia
(c) hydrocarbon ingestion
(d) Goodpasture's syndrome
(e) tuberculosis

I17 Increased density in the metaphyses of the long bones in children occurs in
(a) scurvy
(b) syphilis
(c) mercury poisoning
(d) Caffey's disease
(e) metaphyseal dysostosis

I18 Intrahepatic aneurysms

- (a) are more common than extrahepatic aneurysms of the hepatic artery
- (b) can occur following amphetamine injections
- (c) present as haemobilia in less than one-third of cases
- (d) occur in polyarteritis nodosa
- (e) occur in hereditary telangiectasia

I19 In an adult patient

- (a) a left lateral decubitus abdominal radiograph will demonstrate as little as 10 ml of intraperitoneal air
- (b) an ultrasound examination will show gallstones in about 10% of cases of acute pancreatitis
- (c) gas in the posterior abdominal wall is associated with a penetrating duodenal ulcer
- (d) an elevated serum amylase is diagnostic of acute pancreatitis
- (e) a technetium-99m HIDA scan will confirm acute pancreatitis

I20 In Reiter's syndrome

- (a) involvement of the sacro-iliac joints is usually symmetrical
- (b) there is 'squaring' of the vertebral bodies
- (c) periosteal new bone formation is a characteristic feature
- (d) there can be associated aortic insufficiency
- (e) the joint involvement is frequently associated with concurrent urethritis

I21 Renal papillary necrosis is associated with

- (a) obstructive jaundice
- (b) haemophilia
- (c) thalassaemia
- (d) diabetes mellitus
- (e) polyarteritis nodosa

I22 Meconium ileus

- (a) is associated with microcolon
- (b) usually causes multiple fluid levels on an erect abdominal radiograph
- (c) is associated with diagnostic intraperitoneal calcification on the abdominal radiograph
- (d) occurs most commonly in Down's syndrome
- (e) is caused by the same pathogenic process as a meconium plug

I23 Expansion of the middle cranial fossa is associated with

- (a) chronic subdural haematoma

(b) meningioma
(c) localised hydrocephalus of the temporal horn
(d) Sturge–Weber syndrome
(e) neurofibromatosis

I24 Causes of a cavitating lesion in the chest radiograph are
(a) hamartoma
(b) pulmonary infarction
(c) squamous carcinoma of the bronchus
(d) Caplan's syndrome
(e) haematoma

I25 Motility in the upper third of the oesophagus is decreased in
(a) pseudobulbular palsy
(b) Chagas' disease
(c) myasthenia gravis
(d) scleroderma
(e) cricopharyngeal carcinoma

I26 In Paget's disease
(a) there is increased uptake of radioisotope bone scanning agents in affected areas
(b) internal hydrocephalus is seen
(c) treatment can result in radological improvement
(d) pseudofractures occur on the convex borders of affected long bones
(e) thickening of the iliopectineal line occurs

I27 Cavernous haemangiomas
(a) are the most common benign hepatic tumours
(b) are usually hyperechoic on ultrasound if less than 3 cm in diameter
(c) cause abnormal liver function tests
(d) can develop angiosarcomatous change
(e) on CT show homogeneous opacification after a bolus injection of contrast

I28 In pyogenic osteomyelitis
(a) radiographic changes in the bone are not usually demonstrable before seven days after the onset of symptoms
(b) the first radiographic sign is commonly periosteal new bone formation
(c) the epiphyseal plate acts as barrier to the spread of infection
(d) the adjacent soft tissue planes are displaced
(e) there is calcification of adjacent soft tissue abscesses on healing

I29 Intracranial calcification is seen in
(a) lipoma of corpus callosum

(b) medulloblastoma
(c) cysticercosis
(d) ependymoma
(e) neurofibromatosis

I30 Idiopathic pulmonary haemosiderosis
(a) is associated with fever
(b) is commonly fatal
(c) occurs after 10 years of age
(d) involves the same part of the lung in subsequent attacks
(e) is associated with hilar gland enlargement

I

Answers

I1
(a) **F** adenoma in 90% of cases
(b) **T**
(c) **F** about 30% have stones or nephrocalcinosis
(d) **T** in multiple endocrine neoplasia syndrome
(e) **F** this can also be seen in osteomalacia, Paget's disease myeloma and Cushing's syndrome

I2
(a) **F**
(b) **T**
(c) **F**
(d) **T**
(e) **T**

I3
(a) **T** familial disease
(b) **F** cardiac outline tends to be normal
(c) **F** not inevitable
(d) **T**
(e) **T**

I4
(a) **F** acoustic shadow from fetus causes difficulty in localisation
(b) **F**
(c) **T** 'double bubble' sign
(d) **T** due to fat deposition
(e) **T**

I5
(a) **F**
(b) **T**
(c) **F** effusions are not always present
(d) **F** detection in sputum is difficult. Diagnosis is confirmed by antibody titres
(e) **F** erythromycin

I6
(a) **T**
(b) **T**
(c) **T**

(d) **F** malignant change is to chondrosarcoma
(e) **F** there is usually some new bone formation

I7
(a) **T**
(b) **T** 70% have multiple urinary calculi
(c) **F**
(d) **T** 70–80%. Most frequently *E. coli* or *Proteus*
(e) **F** may simulate a neoplasm or an abscess

I8
(a) **F**
(b) **F**
(c) **T**
(d) **T** occurs typically on diaphragmatic and peri-cardial surfaces
(e) **F**

I9
(a) **T**
(b) **F** sarcoidosis and carcinoma of the bronchus can also cause uptake
(c) **T**
(d) **F** 24 hours later
(e) **T**

I10
(a) **T**
(b) **F**
(c) **F**
(d) **T**
(e) **F**

I11
(a) **F**
(b) **F**
(c) **F** rare unless there is mediastinal lymphadenopathy
(d) **T**
(e) **F**

I12
(a) **F** there is a mild chronic glomerulonephritis leading to renal insufficiency
(b) **T** arise from central area of outer surface of the iliac wing
(c) **T**
(d) **F** small rudimentary patellae may be present
(e) **F** hypoplasia of radial head and capitellum are characteristic

I13
(a) **F**

(b) **T** but less than 2% have bony involvement
(c) **F** no bony changes
(d) **F**
(e) **T** commonest cause of metastases in hands

I14
(a) **F** 80% are opaque
(b) **F** the ducts are thin and irregular
(c) **F** there is dilatation of the duct only as far as the gland
(d) **F** the appearance is normal
(e) **T**

I15
(a) **T**
(b) **T**
(c) **F**
(d) **T**
(e) **T**

I16
(a) **T**
(b) **T**
(c) **T**
(d) **F**
(e) **T**

I17
(a) **T** in the healing process
(b) **T** congenital syphilis
(c) **T**
(d) **F**
(e) **T**

I18
(a) **F**
(b) **T**
(c) **F** 70%
(d) **T**
(e) **F** arteriovenous communication occurs in this disease

I19
(a) **T**
(b) **F** about 70% in the UK
(c) **T**
(d) **F** can be elevated in many acute abdominal conditions
(e) **F** absent activity in gallbladder occurs in acute cholecystitis

I20
(a) **F**

(b) **F** seen in ankylosing spondylitis
(c) **T** particularly in metatarsals and phalanges
(d) **T** late in the course of the disease
(e) **T**

I21
(a) **F**
(b) **F**
(c) **F** seen in sickle cell anaemia
(d) **T**
(e) **T** but very rare

I22
(a) **T**
(b) **F** very viscous, so usually few fluid levels
(c) **F** this is not diagnostic as it follows intrauterine perforation due to any cause
(d) **F** occurs in about 10% of cases of mucoviscidosis
(e) **F** meconium plug seen in premature babies with immature colons

I23
(a) **T**
(b) **F**
(c) **T**
(d) **F**
(e) **T**

I24
(a) **F**
(b) **T**
(c) **T**
(d) **T**
(e) **T**

I25
(a) **T**
(b) **T**
(c) **F**
(d) **F**
(e) **F**

I26
(a) **F** in the sclerotic phase there may be normal activity but the lesion will be obvious on radiographs
(b) **T** due to basilar invagination
(c) **T** with calcitonin and diphosphonates. Improvement appears to be dose related
(d) **T**
(e) **T**

I27
- (a) T
- (b) T
- (c) F   this suggests the lesion may be a metastasis
- (d) F
- (e) F   opacification is not always homogeneous due to thrombus or abnormal haemodynamics

I28
- (a) T
- (b) T
- (c) T
- (d) F   soft tissue planes are obliterated
- (e) F   seen in tuberculosis

I29
- (a) T
- (b) F
- (c) T
- (d) T
- (e) T

I30
- (a) T
- (b) T
- (c) F   before six years of age
- (d) F
- (e) T

J

Questions

J1 Neonatal respiratory distress syndrome
- (a) causes radiographic changes within the first 12 hours
- (b) is associated with reduced surfactant level in the lungs
- (c) is more common in the babies of diabetic mothers
- (d) can cause unilateral change on chest radiograph
- (e) is associated with pneumomediastinum

J2 Unilateral orbital enlargement occurs in
- (a) neurofibromatosis
- (b) carotico-cavernous fistula
- (c) meningioma
- (d) thyrotoxicosis
- (e) rhabdomyosarcoma

J3 Mallet finger
- (a) is caused by avulsion of the flexor digitorum profundus
- (b) is associated with hyperflexion at the proximal interphalangeal joint
- (c) is caused by a flexion force
- (d) can be accompanied by an avulsion fracture
- (e) cannot be excluded on a postero-anterior radiograph

J4 On myelography
- (a) the cervical spinal cord is shown to be expanded in syringomyelia
- (b) intradural extramedullary tumours are shown to cause displacement of the cord
- (c) arteriovenous malformations of the spinal cord are rarely demonstrated
- (d) in spinal dysraphism the position of the conus is best demonstrated in the prone position
- (e) a sequestrated disc fragment can be demonstrated as a filling defect above the affected disc space

J5 Oesophageal atresia
- (a) is commonly associated with prematurity

(b) is not usually associated with other congenital abnormalities
(c) is usually associated with the absence of gas on abdominal radiograph
(d) may cause central cyanosis on feeding
(e) produces pneumonitis particularly in the left lower lobe

J6 Spinal angiomas
(a) are not usually associated with changes on the plain radiograph
(b) most commonly present with subarachnoid haemorrhage
(c) are usually intramedullary
(d) are associated with von Hippel–Lindau disease in 50% of cases
(e) are usually shown on a myelogram in the prone position

J7 Congenital pericardial defects
(a) if incomplete usually occur on the left side of the heart
(b) if complete cause deviation of the heart to the left
(c) are nearly always associated with other congenital cardiothoracic defects
(d) sometimes cause chest pain
(e) if complete cause blurring of the heart outline on the chest radiograph

J8 Caecal volvulus
(a) may occur if the caecum and ileum have a common mesentery
(b) involves rotation of the bowel, commonly more than 180°
(c) is associated with emptiness of the right iliac fossa on an abdominal radiograph
(d) is not accompanied by small bowel fluid levels
(e) is common in Down's syndrome

J9 Sclerosis of vertebral end plates can occur in the following conditions
(a) sarcoidosis
(b) osteopetrosis
(c) rheumatoid arthritis
(d) healing osteomalacia
(e) ankylosing spondylitis

J10 The serum alkaline phosphatase is elevated in
(b) renal osteodystrophy
(b) hyperostosis frontalis interna

(c) pregnancy
(d) osteopetrosis
(e) osteoporosis circumscripta

J11 The following are features of Still's disease:
(a) lymphadenopathy
(b) symmetrical micrognathos
(c) monocytosis
(d) maculopapular rash
(e) periosteal new bone formation

J12 Pneumonia due to *Pneumocystis carinii* in children
(a) occurs most commonly after the age of five years
(b) causes changes on the chest radiograph predominantly in the apices
(c) causes enlargement of the hilar lymph nodes
(d) is associated with pneumomediastinum
(e) progresses to pneumatocoele formation

J13 Widespread patchy sclerosis of the skeleton can be seen in
(a) mast cell reticulosis
(b) carcinoma of the breast
(c) neuroblastoma
(d) fluorosis
(e) myeloid metaplasia

J14 A radiologically demonstrable lipohaemarthrosis can occur with
(a) a fracture of the lateral tibial plateau
(b) a fracture of the radial head
(c) a fracture of the humeral head
(d) rupture of the anterior cruciate ligament
(e) a torn medial meniscus

J15 The following abnormalities suggest childhood non-accidental injury:
(a) metaphyseal fragments
(b) periosteal reactions
(c) fracture of the middle third of the clavicle
(d) fractures of the scapula
(e) chronic subdural haematoma

J16 The following cause lytic lesions in the skull vault:
(a) dystrophia myotonica
(b) Albers–Shönberg disease
(c) craniometaphyseal dysplasia
(d) chordoma
(e) Hand–Schüller–Christian disease

J17 **Persistent bilateral pulmonary changes associated with acute renal failure occur in**
(a) Churg–Strauss syndrome
(b) Goodpasture's syndrome
(c) Wegener's granulomatosis
(d) acute pyelonephritis
(e) systemic lupus erythematosus

J18 **Arteriovenous fistulae can occur in**
(a) renal neoplasms
(b) Sturge–Weber syndrome
(c) a kidney after biopsy
(d) tuberous sclerosis
(e) von Hippel–Lindau disease

J19 **When a bone is fractured**
(a) minimal callus develops if the fragments are impacted
(b) abundant callus is produced if treatment is with internal fixation
(c) non-union is a common occurrence in children
(d) increased activity on a radioisotope bone scan can be present for up to six months after fracture
(e) post-traumatic avascular necrosis can be recognised on the radiograph three weeks after fracture

J20 **The following are seen in a patient with chronic renal failure on haemodialysis:**
(a) abnormalities affecting the ulnar margins of the phalanges
(b) markedly elevated alkaline phosphatase
(c) sclerosis of vertebral end plates
(d) metastatic calcification
(e) periosteal new bone formation

J21 **In a child enlargement of the epiglottis is caused by**
(a) tuberculous infection
(b) *Haemophilus influenzae* infection
(c) chlamydial infection
(d) leukaemic infiltration
(e) respiratory syncytial infection

J22 **Concavity of the vertebral body end plates occurs in**
(a) Morquio–Brailsford dystrophy
(b) osteogenesis imperfecta
(c) sickle cell disease
(d) thalassaemia
(e) brucellosis

J23 Mitral subvalvular calcification
(a) is seen on the lateral chest radiograph above a line joining the tracheal bifurcation and the anterior sterno-diaphragmatic angle
(b) is caused by rheumatic fever
(c) occurs in association with Marfan's syndrome
(d) can cause symptoms of mitral stenosis
(e) is associated with atrio-ventricular conduction defects

J24 Vitamin C deficiency causes
(a) a zone of translucency on the diaphyseal side of the epiphysis in infants
(b) produces osteoporosis in the adult
(c) tenderness of the lower limbs in children
(d) calcific subperiosteal haematoma
(e) ill-defined epiphyses in infants

J25 When there has been trauma to the skull
(a) on a anteroposterior radiograph lateral displacement of the calcified pineal greater than 2 mm is significant
(b) a linear fracture crossing a dural sinus is associated with an extradural haematoma
(c) depression of the skull can occur in neonates without fracture
(d) subdural haematomas are associated with skull fracture in 90% of cases
(e) a fracture involving a paranasal sinus is associated with pneumocephalus is about 10% of cases

J26 In the congenital rubella syndrome the following occur:
(a) atrial septal defects
(b) cataracts
(c) rudimentary epiphyses
(d) asplenia
(e) congenital dislocation of the shoulder

J27 Osteogenesis imperfecta
(a) can be diagnosed in utero
(b) is inherited as an autosomal dominant
(c) can be complicated by deafness
(d) is associated with metaphyseal fractures
(e) is associated with non-union of fractures

J28 In a duplex kidney
(a) the ureter draining the lower moiety is more prone to reflux
(b) the ureter draining the upper moiety enters the bladder above that draining the lower moiety

- (c) there is a high incidence of malrotation
- (d) the upper moiety is more likely to be associated with an ectopic ureterocoele
- (e) and ectopic ureter there is likely to be associated enuresis in the male

J29 The Eisenmenger syndrome
- (a) with a ventricular septal defect produces little enlargement of the pulmonary trunk
- (b) is commonly associated with a reduction in cardiac size with the onset of cyanosis
- (c) is not associated with patent ductus arteriosus
- (d) is not associated with secondary polycythemia
- (e) is associated with asplenia

J30 Duplication cysts
- (a) can cause a mass in the posterior mediastinum
- (b) always communicate with the alimentary canal
- (c) present with malabsorption
- (d) can contain gastric mucosa
- (e) occur in association with mucoviscidosis

J

Answers

J1
(a) **T** there are always radiographic changes within 12 hours
(b) **T**
(c) **T**
(d) **F** bilateral, symmetrical change
(e) **T**

J2
(a) **T**
(c) **T**
(c) **T**
(d) **F**
(e) **T**

J3
(a) **F** avulsion of the extensor tendon at its insertion on the dorsal surface of the distal phalanx
(b) **F**
(c) **T** forcible flexion of the distal phalanx while the extensor is taut
(d) **T**
(e) **T**

J4
(a) **T**
(b) **T**
(c) **F** usually shown
(d) **F** supine position
(e) **T**

J5
(a) **T**
(b) **F** other congenital abnormalities occur in greater than 50%. Cardiovascular, gastrointestinal and genitourinary
(c) **F**
(d) **T**
(e) **F** right upper lobe

J6
(a) **T**

(b) **F** most present with cord compression
(c) **F**
(d) **F** about 15%
(d) **F** the majority are on the dorsum of the cord
          and best demonstrated in the supine position

J7
(a) **T**
(b) **T**
(c) **F** only 20%. Patent ductus arteriosus, atrial
          septal defect, bronchogenic cyst
(d) **T** due to torsion of the great arteries
(e) **T** due to increased mobility of the heart

J8
(a) **T**
(b) **T** 180–360°
(c) **T**
(d) **F** this is true of signoid volvulus
(e) **F**

J9
(a) **T**
(b) **T**
(c) **F**
(d) **T**
(e) **F**

J10
(a) **T**
(b) **F**
(c) **T**
(d) **F**
(e) **T**

J11
(a) **T**
(b) **T**
(c) **F** leucopenia
(d) **T**
(e) **T** affects metacarpals, metatarsals and phalanges

J12
(a) **F** most commonly occurs in premature and
          unwell infants
(b) **F** usually bilateral central shadowing with
          sparing of the apices and periphery of the lungs
(c) **F**
(d) **T** in association with interstitial emphysema
(e) **F**

J13
(a) **T**

(b) **T**
(c) **F**
(d) **T**
(e) **T**

J14
(a) **T**
(b) **T**
(c) **T**
(d) **F**
(e) **F**

J15
(a) **T** due to epiphyseal separation
(b) **T** occur commonly along the whole diaphysis and involve the metaphysis
(d) **F**
(d) **T**
(e) **T**

J16
(a) **F** thick skull, large frontal sinuses with small pituitary fossa
(b) **F** marble bone disease
(c) **F** thickening of the occipital and frontal bones
(d) **F**
(e) **T**

J17
(a) **T** patients usually have allergic diathesis. Resembles polyarteritis nodosa
(b) **T** type 2 allergic reaction involving basement membrane of the kidney and lungs
(c) **T** lung involvement invariable, but renal involvement not seen in milder cases
(d) **F**
(e) **T**

J18
(a) **T**
(b) **T**
(c) **T**
(d) **F**
(e) **T**

J19
(a) **T**
(b) **F**
(c) **F** this suggests movement at the fracture site or infection
(d) **T** activity can be increased for up to 18 months
(e) **F** unusual to see any change before two months

J20
(a) **F** radial margins affected
(b) **F** usually normal or slightly elevated
(c) **T**
(d) **T**
(e) **T**

J21
(a) **F**
(b) **T**
(c) **F**
(d) **F**
(e) **F**

J22
(a) **F**
(b) **T**
(c) **T** infarcts of vertebral bodies cause end-plate depression
(d) **F** diffuse demineralisation occurs but vertebral collapse is very uncommon
(e) **F**

J23
(a) **F** the mitral valve lies below this line
(b) **F** seen in old age
(c) **T** there is calcification and dilatation of the annulus
(d) **F** mitral regurgitation
(e) **T** occur when calcium is deposited in the conduction system

J24
(a) **T**
(b) **T**
(c) **T**
(d) **T** calcification occurs especially on treatment
(e) **F** well-defined

J25
(a) **T** however, the pineal may be central with bilateral subdural haematoma
(b) **F** this is associated with venous thrombosis
(c) **T**
(d) **F** about 50% of cases
(e) **T**

J26
(a) **F**
(b) **T**
(c) **F** metaphyses
(d) **F** splenomegaly
(e) **T**

J27
(a) **T**
(b) **T** with variable penetrance
(c) **T**
(d) **F**
(e) **F** fractures unite with the production of abundant callus

J28
(a) **T**
(b) **F**
(c) **T**
(d) **T**
(e) **F** in the male the ureter opens above the external sphincter

J29
(a) **T**
(b) **T**
(c) **F**
(d) **F**
(e) **F**

J30
(a) **T** arise from the oesophagus, duodenum and jejunum and can extend through the diaphragm
(b) **F** most do not
(c) **F** normally present as intestinal obstruction, an abdominal mass, haematemesis or melaena
(d) **T**
(e) **F**

Bibliography

Below is a list of the texts from which the majority of questions have been verified.

Baddely, Nolan and Salmon 1978 *Radiological Atlas of Biliary and Pancreatic Disease*. HM & M Publishers Ltd, Aylesbury

Caffey J 1978 *Paediatric X-Ray Diagnosis*. Year Book Medical Publishers, London Chicago

Cosgrove D O and McCready V R 1982 *Ultrasound Imaging*. John Wiley and Sons, Chichester New York

Du Boulay G H 1965 *Principles of X-Ray Diagnosis of the Skull*. Butterworths, London Boston

Ed. Emerson P *Thoracic Medicine*. Butterworths, London Boston

Felson B 1973 *Chest Roentgenology*. W B Saunders Company, Philadelphia London Toronto

Freiberger R H and Kaye J J 1979 *Arthography*. Appleton-Century-Crofts, New York

Gordon I R S and Ross F G M 1977 *Diagnostic Radiology in Paediatrics*. Butterworths, London Boston

Hoeffken W and Lanyi M 1977 *Mammography*. W B Saunders Company, Philadelphia, London Toronto. Georg Thieme Publishers, Stuttgart

Husband J E and Kelsey Fry I 1981 *Computed Tomography of the Body*. Macmillan, London

Ed. Isselbacher K J, Adams R D, Braunwald E, Petersdorf R J and Wilson J D 1980 *Harrison's Principles of Internal Medicine*. McGraw Hill International Book Company, London Dordrecht Boston

Jefferson K and Rees R 1973 *Clinical Cardiac Radiology*. Butterworths, London Toronto

Laufer I 1979 *Double Contrast Gastrointestinal Radiology*. W B Saunders Company, Philadelphia London Toronto

Lodwick G S 1971 *The Bones and Joints*. Year Book Medical Publishers, Chicago

Maisey M 1980 *Nuclear Medicine*. Update Books

Marshak R H and Lindner A E 1976 *Radiology of the Small Intestine*. W S Saunders Company, Philadelphia London Toronto

Murray R O and Jacobson H G 1971 *The Radiology of Skeletal Disorders*. Churchill Livingstone, Edinburgh

Rogers L F 1982 *Radiology of Skeletal Trauma*. Churchill Livingstone, Edinburgh

Samuel F and Lloyd G A S 1978 *Clinical Radiology of the Ear, Nose and Throat*. H K Lewis and Co Ltd, London

Shapiro R 1975 *Myelography*. Year Book Medical Publishers, Chicago

Sherwood T, Davidson A J and Talner L B 1980 *Uroradiology*. Blackwell Scientific Publications, Edinburgh

Sutton D 1980 *A Textbook of Radiology and Imaging*. Churchill Livingstone, Edinburgh